Highlights in the History

of the

Army Nurse Corps

Highlights in the History of the Army Nurse Corps

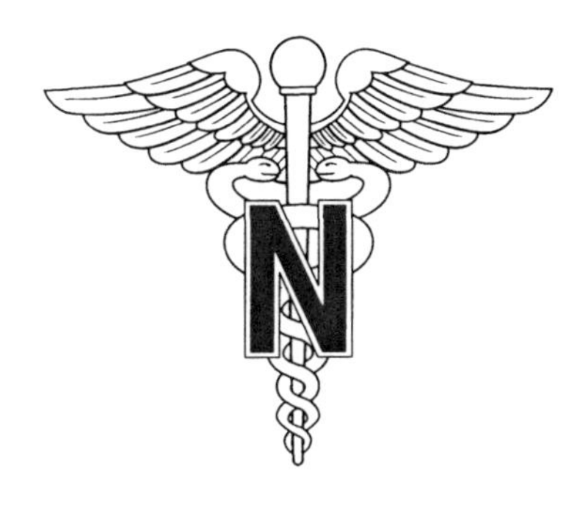

University Press of the Pacific
Honolulu . Hawaii

Highlights in the History of the
Army Nurse Corps

Edited by
Carolyn M. Feller
Constance J. Moore

ISBN:0-89875-493-3

Reprinted from the 1995 edition

University Press of the Pacific
Honolulu, Hawaii
http://www.universitypressofthepacific.com

FOREWORD

Throughout its history, the Army Nurse Corps has evolved as a world-class center of excellence for military nursing and a bench mark for caring for the entire nursing community. Army nurses have remained at the forefront of change, providing leadership in integrating nursing research and nursing education into clinical practice. Today, we continue the legacy of a proud heritage by maintaining the highest standards of professionalism in nursing and in military service. Our professional evolution reflects not only the changing requirements of a progressive Army, but also our expanding roles in supporting the health care needs of our nation. While endeavoring to meet the contemporary challenges posed by changes in the military mission, organizational structures, technological advances, and increased services, we have kept our commitment to support the health care needs of the soldier, the family, and other beneficiaries. Our past has prepared us to meet the challenges of today and validates our potential for meeting the health care challenges of the future. The global nature of our mission provides Army nursing the unique opportunity to serve both country and humanity. I am proud to join the thousands of nurses who are now a part of this great history, and I share in the excitement and expectations of accomplishments yet to come. These highlights of our past provide testimony to our heritage and our professional contributions to the Army Medical Department, the Army, and the nation. It is these very contributions of each member of the Corps that demonstrate that Army nurses not only serve proudly but are leaders in caring as they serve.

NANCY R. ADAMS
Brigadier General, ANC
Chief, Army Nurse Corps

PREFACE

This publication chronicles the major events in the proud history of the Army Nurse Corps. Although it is not intended as an analysis of historical events, it highlights the major milestones in the evolution of the Corps. The notable contributions of Corps members and their colleagues to military and civilian nursing practice, education, administration, and research are recorded. Legislation and other significant events that effected changes in the history of the Corps are mentioned. Emphasis is placed on the continuing efforts of the Corps to provide high-quality nursing care to soldiers, their families, and retired military and their dependents in time of peace and war and in the carrying out of humanitarian missions. Although not every Corps member is mentioned, all the entries reflect the proud heritage of the Corps and provide ideas for scholarly historical research. History provides a basis for the present and direction for the future. At the present time, numerous changes in the military and the worldwide community are creating new and complex challenges for the Corps. Chiefs of the Army Nurse Corps, past and present, have provided professional and committed leadership to prepare us for these challenges.

This chronology was first prepared in 1959, with revisions in 1960, 1961, 1973, 1975, 1981, and 1987. Although the original format is preserved, the entire manuscript has been updated and new appendixes added. John Birmingham of the Center of Military History's Office of Production Services reformatted the text. Catherine A. Heerin edited and, with the assistance of Joycelyn M. Canery, proofread the manuscript. The authors alone are responsible for errors and omissions.

Washington, D.C.

CAROLYN M. FELLER
Lieutenant Colonel, ANC, USAR

CONSTANCE J. MOORE
Major, ANC

CONTENTS

Highlights in the History of the Army Nurse Corps

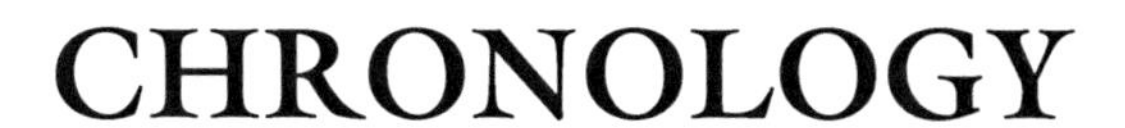

CHRONOLOGY

CHRONOLOGY

14 Jun 1775 The Second Continental Congress authorized the Continental Army which later became the United States Army. Shortly thereafter, Maj. Gen. Horatio Gates in the northern frontier reported to Commander in Chief George Washington that "the sick suffered much for Want of good female Nurses." General Washington then asked the Congress for "a matron to supervise the nurses, bedding, etc.," and for nurses "to attend the sick and obey the matron's orders."

27 Jul 1775 The Second Continental Congress authorized medical support for a Continental Army of 20,000 men, and submitted a plan to General Washington for creating "an Hospital" (a Medical Department). This plan provided one nurse for every ten patients and "that a matron be allotted to every hundred sick or wounded, who shall take care that the provisions are properly prepared; that the wards, beds, and utensils be kept in neat order; and that the most exact economy be observed in her department."

Although the women who tended the sick and wounded during the Revolutionary War were not nurses as known in the modern sense, they helped blaze the trail for another generation nearly one hundred years later, in 1873, when civilian hospitals in America began operating recognized schools of nursing.

7 Apr 1777 The pay of the nurse, originally $2 a month and one ration per day, was increased to $8 per month and one ration per day. The matron received $15 per month and a daily ration.

1783–1817 After the Revolutionary War (1775–1783), the Congress drastically reduced the size of the military establishment. Medical service was provided at regimental level for the separate garrisons of a small, scattered Army during this period. Patient care was performed by soldiers detailed from the companies. There was no centralized medical direction by a formally organized medical department until the War of 1812.

14 Apr 1818 The Medical Department was reestablished by the Congress as a continuing staff agency under the direction of a Surgeon General, Dr Joseph Lovell The passage of the Army Reorganization Act of 1818 marked the beginning of the modern Medical Department of the United States Army.

Aug 1856 The Secretary of War was authorized to appoint enlisted men as hospital stewards, equivalent to noncommissioned officers.

10 Jun 1861 Two months after the Civil War began on 12 April 1861, the Secretary of War appointed Dorothea Lynde Dix, famed for her work on behalf of the mentally ill, as Superintendent of Women Nurses for the Union Army. Despite the impressive title, Miss Dix's authority was vague and limited: "to select and assign women nurses to general or permanent military hospitals, they not to be employed in such hospitals without her sanction and approval except in cases of urgent need." Miss Dix headed the list of about six thousand women who served the federal forces. Some of the women, before reporting for assignment, received a short course in nursing under the dedicated direction of Dr. Elizabeth Blackwell, the first woman to receive a medical degree in the United States.

3 Aug 1861 The Congress authorized The Surgeon General to employ women as nurses for Army hospitals at a salary of $12 per month plus one ration.

1861–1865 During the Civil War (12 April 1861–26 May 1865), many women served as nurses in the hospitals of both the Union and the Confederate Armies, among them a large number of Catholic sisters of several religious orders. Some of the women who served in the Union hospitals were not on the Army payroll but were sponsored by the United States Sanitary Commission or by volunteer agencies. Women served as nurses in many hospitals, but the work was largely limited to preparing diets, supervising the distribution of supplies furnished by volunteer groups, and housekeeping details. Nonetheless, nearly one hundred years before development of the mid-twentieth century concept of progressive patient care, one nurse wrote of separating patients according to their needs:

> "My ward was now divided into three rooms; and, under favor of the matron, had managed to sort out the patients in such a way that I had what I called my 'duty room,' my 'pleasure room,' and my 'pathetic room,' and worked for each in a different way. One, I visited with a dressing tray full of rollers, plasters, and pins; another, with books, flowers, games, and gossips, a third, with teapots, lullabies, consolation and—sometimes—a shroud."
>
> Louisa May Alcott
> *Hospital Sketches*, 1863

1865–1898 Following the Civil War, soldiers continued to perform patient care duties in Army hospitals. On 1 March 1887, the Congress established a Hospital Corps (24 Stat. 435) consisting of enlisted hospital stewards and privates as a part of the Army Medical Department. Since these soldiers were permanently assigned to the Medical Department, training programs were developed in the various needed skills, including nursing functions. Thus began the formal establishment of a career for enlisted personnel in the Medical Department. In 1891, Capt. John Van Renssalaer Hoff, MC, organized the first company of instruction for members of the Hospital Corps at Fort Riley, Kansas.

28 Apr 1898 At the onset of the Spanish-American War, the Surgeon General requested and promptly received congressional authority to appoint women nurses under contract at the rate of $30 per month and a daily ration.

Dr. Anita Newcomb McGee, Vice President of the National Society of the Daughters of the American Revolution (DAR), was placed in charge of selecting graduate nurses for the Army. Military nursing had been almost dormant since the Civil War. Dr. McGee suggested that the DAR act as an application review board for military nursing services. Thus the DAR Hospital Corps was founded, with Dr. McGee as its director. Civilian hospitals had been operating schools of nursing since 1873. Dr. McGee set high standards for volunteer applicants. For the most part, only graduates certified by approval of nursing school directors were accepted for appointment under contract to the Army. Many of the nurses were of the religious orders Sisters of Charity, Sisters of Mercy, and Sisters of the Holy Cross. Other nurses were obtained through the assistance of the Red Cross Society for the Maintenance of Trained Nurses in New York. Military nursing achieved a high level of professional competence. These military nurses became known as "contract nurses" of the Army.

Jul 1898 Between May and July, almost twelve hundred nurses had volunteered. The emergency which made the nursing services of women acceptable resulted from the inability of the Army Medical Department to enlist within a few weeks six thousand or more men qualified by previous experience to perform important patient care duties and from the epidemic prevalence of typhoid fever in the Army's camps. One nurse in a field hospital in Coamo, Puerto Rico, wrote:

> "The nurses quartered in an old Spanish house in Coamo, located in a banana grove. We drove to camp in mule ambulances. Put in long hours.... Sick men from 3rd Wisconsin, 16th Pennsylvania, and 3rd Kentucky Regiments cared for by Army Nurses. All water for any purpose hauled in barrels from a spring more than a mile away. Tents crowded,

typhoid fever, dysentery and diarrhea, conditions bad, no ice, no diet kitchen."

1898–1901 Slightly more than fifteen hundred women nurses signed governmental contracts. Contract nurses served in the United States, Cuba, Puerto Rico, the Philippine Islands, Hawaii, China, briefly in Japan, and on the hospital ship *Relief.* The maximum number on duty was 1,563 on 15 September 1898.

After the Spanish-American War ended with the signing of the Peace Protocol on 12 August 1898, and as soon as the typhoid epidemic in the United States was brought under control in 1899, the number of women nurses was reduced to 700. By June 1900, there were 210 nurses serving under contract with the Army.

During and following the Spanish-American War, fifteen nurses died of typhoid fever. Another, Clara Louise Maass of New Jersey, died of yellow fever on 24 August 1901. A former contract nurse, Miss Maass was not connected with the experiments of the Yellow Fever Commission (a board headed by Maj. Walter Reed, MC), but volunteered as a subject in the research on modes of transmission of the disease while she was employed in Cuba at the Las Animas Hospital, Havana. In 1904, William C. Gorgas, MC (later the Surgeon General, 1914–1918), who put the U.S. Army research findings to practical use in Cuba and later in Panama, stated that Miss Maass' death was a contributing factor in convincing physicians and the public that yellow fever was in fact transmitted by a mosquito vector.

29 Aug 1898 The Surgeon General established a Nurse Corps Division in his office to direct and coordinate the efforts of military nursing. Dr. McGee was appointed Acting Assistant Surgeon and placed in charge. She immediately set about to make military nursing an attractive career.

20 Jun 1899 The first Army regulations governing the Nurse Corps were published as a circular, approved by the Secretary of War and issued from the Surgeon General's Office. These regulations governed the appointment of nurses and defined their duties, pay, and privileges. Quarters and rations, transportation expenses, leave of absence in the proportion of thirty days for each year of past service, care when sick, a uniform, and a badge were authorized for the nurse. The pay was increased to $40 a month in the United States and to $50 in overseas areas. The regulations were reissued on 9 March 1900, with but two important changes: appointments were limited to citizens of the United States; and the annual leave was changed to thirty days authorized in each calendar year, regardless of length of service.

1901 A bill came before the Congress to establish a permanent Nurse Corps. While most contract nurses had been subject to Army control and regulations, others had been paid by private sources and were thus under the control of private individuals and voluntary organizations, such as the DAR and the Red Cross Societies. Such an arrangement created difficult administrative problems. This, coupled with the recognized need for women nurses, made it imperative that the status of the Army nurse be clarified and officially regulated. Earlier, Surgeon General George M. Sternberg had not been fully convinced that a permanent Nurse Corps should be established. He had been reluctant to have women serve with the troops in the field; he had commented on the added expense of "luxuries" for the women such as bureaus, rocking chairs, and other special items not previously requisitioned for the men; and many of his senior medical officers had disapproved of the idea. However, the record of service of the women nurses who served during the Spanish-American War was the convincing factor and paved the way for establishment of a permanent Nurse Corps. The Surgeon General, in his annual report of 1899, said:

> "American women may well feel proud of the record made by these nurses in 1898–99, for every medical officer with whom they served has testified to their intelligence, and skill, their earnestness, devotion and self-sacrifice."

At the request of Surgeon General Sternberg, Dr. McGee wrote a bill to establish a Nurse Corps (female). What she wrote eventually became Section 19 of the Army Reorganization Act of 1901. Congress passed the bill after Dr. McGee left office on 31 December 1900, but she became known as the "Founder of the Army Nurse Corps."

2 Feb 1901 The Nurse Corps (female) became a permanent corps of the Medical Department under the Army Reorganization Act (31 Stat. 753) passed by the Congress. Nurses were *appointed* in the Regular Army for a three-year period, although nurses were not actually *commissioned* as officers in the Regular Army until forty-six years later—on 16 April 1947. The appointment could be renewed provided the applicant had a "satisfactory record for efficiency, conduct and health." (The application for continuance of service every three years was discontinued in 1934.) The law directed the Surgeon General to maintain a list of qualified nurses who were willing to serve in an emergency. Therefore, provision was made to appoint a certain number of nurses with at least six months of satisfactory service in the Army on a reserve status. This was the first Reserve Corps authorized in the Army Medical Department. (The Army Medical Reserve Corps for medical officers only, 35 Stat. 66, forerunner of today's reserve component, was established by the Congress on 23 April 1908.) Each reserve nurse signed an agreement to enter active service whenever required and to report by letter to the Surgeon General every six months. There were thirty-seven reserve nurses who wore the badge of the Army nurse

28 Feb 1901 The number of "charter" members of the Nurse Corps as of this date was generally considered to be 202. There were actually 220 nurses on active duty, but this number included those at home awaiting discharge. By 1 July, 176 nurses remained in the Corps.

15 Mar 1901 Dita H. Kinney, a former contract nurse, was officially appointed the first Superintendent of the Corps, a position she had held since 1 January 1901. Mrs. Kinney served as Superintendent of the Corps until she resigned on 31 July 1909.

1902 The authorized strength of the Nurse Corps was fixed at 100 nurses and remained unchanged for ten years.

12 Aug 1909 Jane A. Delano, a graduate nurse and active Red Cross worker, was appointed Superintendent of the Corps. She resigned on 31 March 1912 to serve as Chairman of the American Red Cross Nursing Service. In 1911, during Miss Delano's tenure as Superintendent of the Corps, the enrolled nurses of the American Red Cross were designated as the primary source of reserve nurses for the Army. The "reserve list" provision in the basic law had attracted few nurses in a decade of effort, but by 30 June 1913, there were 4,000 nurses eligible, by their consent, for active military duty assignment.

1912–1914 The authorized strength of the Nurse Corps was increased to 125 in 1912 and to 150 in 1914.

1 Apr 1912 Isabel McIsaac was appointed Superintendent of the Corps and served until her death on 21 September 1914.

22 Sep 1914 Dora E. Thompson was appointed the fourth Superintendent of the Corps. Miss Thompson was the first Regular Army nurse to serve as Superintendent.

6 Apr 1917 The United States entered World War I. There were 403 nurses on active duty, including 170 reserve nurses who had been ordered to duty (as a result of incidents on the Mexican border) in twelve Army hospitals in Texas, Arizona, and New Mexico. By 30 June 1917, there were 1,176 nurses on duty. One year later, 12,186 nurses (2,000 Regular Army and 10,186 reserve) were on active duty serving at 198 stations worldwide.

May 1917 Six base (general) hospitals, with more than four hundred nurses, sailed for France for service with the British Expeditionary Forces. Two nurses with Base Hospital No. 12, Mercy and Wesley Memorial Hospitals, Chicago, Illinois, were killed en route by brass fragments caused by the faulty discharge of a gun. These hospitals were the first organized Army forces to serve in France in World War I. On 2 October 1917, General John J. Pershing sent a cabled request "for a competent member of the Nurse Corps" to supervise nursing activities in the American Expeditionary Forces (AEF). Bessie S. Bell, then Chief Nurse of Walter Reed General Hospital, reported to serve on 13 November 1917.

25 May 1918 The Army School of Nursing was authorized by the Secretary of War as an alternative to utilizing nurses' aides in Army hospitals. Courses of instruction opened at several Army hospitals in July 1918. Annie W. Goodrich, who had been appointed under contract as Chief Inspector Nurse for the Army, became the first Dean of the Army School of Nursing. (On 23 March 1923, she was awarded the Distinguished Service Medal.) Although the Adjutant General authorized a military uniform and an insignia consisting of a bronze lamp superimposed on the caduceus, the students in the Army School of Nursing retained civilian status. In December 1918 there were 1,578 students in the school. No decision had been made concerning the continuance of the school after the war. In February 1919 the Surgeon General gave assurance that the school would be continued. Of the students who elected to continue, 508 completed the course. By 1923, the school had been consolidated at Walter Reed General Hospital. It was discontinued by the Secretary of War on 12 August 1931 as an economy measure. A total of 937 young women completed the course in nursing and received the diploma of the school. Among its many illustrious graduates were Mary G. Phillips and Ruby F. Bryant, who later became Chiefs of the Army Nurse Corps. Other well-known graduates include Margaret Tracy '21, Lulu Wolf Hassenplug '24, Virginia Henderson '21, Myrtle Hodgkins Coe '27, Marion Kalkman '31, Edith Haydon '21, Laura Wood Fitzsimmons '26, Laura Louise Baker '21, Ruth Hubbard '21, Gertrude Wahl Small '21, Ann Louise Finch '21, Bossie Bell Randle '21, Eleanor L. Kennedy Berchtold '21, and Portia Irick '26. The list of achievers is extensive; many others directed nursing services in hospitals or agencies or were university faculty members. *The Lamp and the Caduceus*, written by Marlette Conde and published by the Army School of Nursing Alumnae Association in 1975, is a very interesting and authentic account of the beginning, progress, and closing of the Army School of Nursing.

30 Jun 1918 Of the 12,186 nurses on active duty, 5,350 were serving overseas.

9 Jul 1918 The Nurse Corps (female) was redesignated the Army Nurse Corps by the Army Reorganization Act of 1918. The 1918 act (40 Stat. 879) restricted appointments to women nurses. Base pay was increased to $60 per month.

11 Nov 1918 Armistice Day. During World War I, the peak strength of the Army Nurse Corps reached 21,480 on 11 November 1918. More than ten thousand nurses had served in overseas areas in France, Belgium, England, Italy, and Serbia, as well as in Siberia, Hawaii, Puerto Rico, and the Philippines. Included were ten Sisters of Charity who served with Base Hospital No. 102 in Vicenza, Italy. Army nurses were assigned to casualty clearing stations and surgical teams in field hospitals as well as to mobile, evacuation, base, camp, and convalescent hospitals. They also served on hospital trains and transport ships. (Following the Armistice, nurses served with the occupation forces in Germany until the American forces were returned in 1923.)

Several nurses were wounded, but none died as a result of enemy action. There were, however, more than two hundred deaths largely caused by influenza and pneumonia. The Distinguished Service Cross (second in rank only to the Medal of Honor, the highest decoration in combat) was awarded to 3 Army nurses. The Distinguished Service Medal (highest decoration in noncombat) was awarded to 23 Army nurses. In addition to other United States Army decorations, 28 Army nurses were awarded the French Croix de Guerre, 69 the British Royal Red Cross, and 2 the British Military Medal. Many Army nurses were named in British Army dispatches for their meritorious service.

Nurses who remained in the United States served with distinction in busy cantonment and general hospitals, at ports of embarkation, and at other military outposts. Many were cited for meritorious service.

13 Nov 1918 Eighteen African American nurses were assigned to duty in the ANC following the influenza epidemic. Nine were assigned to Camp Grant, Illinois, and nine to Camp Sherman, Ohio. Their living quarters were separate, but they were assigned to duties in an integrated hospital. By August 1919 the reduction in force necessitated their release.

15 Apr 1919 Jane A. Delano, Chairman of the Red Cross Nursing Service and former Superintendent of the Army Nurse Corps, died in an Army hospital in France (Base Hospital No. 69 at Savenay). She had been making an official visit to review the activities of the American Red Cross. Miss Delano was buried at Loire, France, with military honors and was awarded the Distinguished Service Medal posthumously. Her body was reinterred in the nurses' plot in Arlington National Cemetery in 1920, and Delano Hall, until recently a residence for nurses and nursing students at Walter Reed Army Medical Center, was named in her honor.

29 Dec 1919 Dora E. Thompson, a recipient of the Distinguished Service Medal for her leadership of the Corps during World War I, resigned as

Superintendent of the Army Nurse Corps, but accepted reappointment as Assistant Superintendent. Miss Thompson held the relative rank of captain after July 1920 and served with distinction until she retired on 31 August 1932, after more than thirty years of active service.

30 Dec 1919 Julia C. Stimson, a graduate of Vassar College and New York Hospital School of Nursing, became the fifth Superintendent of the Army Nurse Corps. Miss Stimson had been Chief Nurse of one of the base hospitals that served the British Expeditionary Forces. In March 1918, she became Chief of the Red Cross Nursing Service in France and, on 15 November 1918, the Director of Nursing Service, American Expeditionary Forces, France. In July 1919, she succeeded Annie W. Goodrich as Dean, Army School of Nursing. After appointment as Superintendent of the Army Nurse Corps, Miss Stimson held both positions until the Army School of Nursing closed on 31 January 1933. In 1921, she was awarded an honorary degree of Doctor of Science by Mount Holyoke College.

4 Jun 1920 An Army Reorganization Act authorized relative rank for Army nurses. The act was passed by the Congress in recognition of the outstanding services of more than twenty thousand Army nurses during World War I. It authorized granting of the status of an officer with relative rank to Army nurses from second lieutenant through major:

> "and as regards medical and sanitary matters and all other work within the line of their professional duties [they] shall have authority in and about military hospitals next after officers of the Medical Department. The Secretary of War shall make the necessary regulations prescribing the rights and privileges conferred by such relative rank."

Although the act allowed Army nurses to wear the insignia of the relative rank, the Secretary of War did not prescribe full rights and privileges, such as base pay, for nurses equal to that of an officer of comparable grade.

30 Jun 1921 Demobilization had reduced the Army Nurse Corps to 851 nurses with the following relative ranks: 1 major, 4 captains, 74 first lieutenants, and 772 second lieutenants.

Apr 1923 Annie W. Goodrich, former Chief Inspecting Nurse for the Army and the first Dean of the Army School of Nursing, was appointed Dean of the Yale School of Nursing—the first university-based undergraduate school of nursing.

13 May 1926 Nurses were authorized retirement on length of service.

Jul 1929 Maj. Julia C. Stimson was awarded the Florence Nightingale Medal in recognition of her service as Chief of the Red Cross Nursing Service in France and her service in the American Expeditionary Forces. This medal is a memorial to Miss Nightingale and is awarded by the International Committee of the Red Cross to honor those who have given distinguished and devoted service to the sick and wounded in times of war and peace and in disasters through service or education.

20 Jun 1930 Retirement for disability incurred in the line of duty with no minimum length of service requirement was authorized for nurses.

1937 Reid Hall, a residence for members of the Army Nurse Corps at the Station Hospital, Fort Sam Houston, Texas, was named in memory of Capt. Elizabeth D. Reid, ANC. Captain Reid had served in the Army with conspicuous distinction for twenty-nine years before her retirement in 1935. Captain Reid died in 1936.

31 May 1937 Maj. Julia C. Stimson retired after twenty years of service—seventeen as Superintendent of the Army Nurse Corps. She served as President of the American Nurses' Association from 1938 to 1944 and as Chairman of the Nursing Council on National Defense, which was later renamed National Nursing Council for War Service, from July 1940 to July 1942, and as a member thereafter. Major Stimson served on active duty from 7 October 1942 to 14 April 1943 to publicize the need for nurses in the armed services. Based on her service during World War II, she was advanced to the grade of colonel on the retired list on 13 August 1948 as a result of Public Law 810, 80th Congress. Colonel Stimson died a few weeks later on 30 September 1948.

1 Jun 1937 Maj. Julia O. Flikke became the sixth Superintendent of the Army Nurse Corps.

8 Nov 1938 The "Spirit of Nursing" monument, a symbolic figure carved from Tennessee marble by Miss Frances Rich, was dedicated. This monument marks the plot reserved for military nurses in Arlington National Cemetery.

8 Sep 1939 A state of Limited Emergency was declared because of the war in Europe. There were 625 Regular Army nurses on active duty. The authorized strength of the Army Nurse Corps (Regular) was immediately increased to 949.

30 Jun 1940 There were 942 Regular Army nurses in the Corps. An additional 15,770 nurses, enrolled in the First Reserve of the American Red Cross Nursing Service, were presumably available for service if needed.

27 May 1941 A state of National Emergency was declared because of the threat of global war. Once again, it became necessary to activate reserve nurses.

7 Dec 1941 Japanese planes bombed Pearl Harbor. Within forty-eight hours, the United States was formally at war with Japan, Germany, and Italy. There were fewer than seven thousand Army nurses on active duty when the United States entered World War II. Six months later, there were more than twelve thousand nurses on active duty.

1942 Lt. Della Raney was selected as the first African American Chief Nurse in the ANC while serving at Tuskegee Air Field, Alabama. Approximately five hundred black nurses served in the Army Nurse Corps during World War II. They served in segregated units in the United States as well as overseas. First Lt. Susan Freeman was chief of the thirty nurses of the 25th Station Hospital that arrived at Roberts Field, Liberia, in March 1943. Lieutenant Freeman was awarded the Ribbon of the Knight Official, Liberian Order of African Redemption, when her tour of duty ended. In 1944, she was promoted to the rank of captain and presented the Mary Mahoney Award by the National Association of Colored Graduate Nurses for her service during the Ohio flood disaster and in recognition of being the first black nurse to command an overseas unit in the ANC. First Lt. Agnes B. Glass was the Chief Nurse of the 335th Station Hospital at Tagap, Burma, that opened in late December 1944. During World War II, a total of 512 African American nurses were in the Army Nurse Corps: 9 were in the grade of captain, 115 were first lieutenants, and 388 were second lieutenants.

13 Mar 1942 Maj. Julia O. Flikke, Superintendent of the Army Nurse Corps, received a temporary commission as a colonel in the AUS (Army of the United States). Her assistant, Capt. Florence A. Blanchfield, received a temporary commission in the grade of lieutenant colonel, AUS. Although they wore the insignia of their grade, they were denied the pay of that grade, a decision of the Comptroller General which stated that these women were not "persons" in the sense of the law under which they were promoted. (In 1952, the 82d Congress in Private Law 716 reversed the decision and they, then retired, received the pay which had been withheld for ten years.)

9 Apr 1942 The fall of Bataan. From December until early April, the fighting forces, including doctors, nurses, and corpsmen alike, had endured relentless hardships. On the night of 8 April, the remaining forces were ordered to withdraw to Corregidor as Bataan was falling. At Corregidor, Lt. Gen. Jonathan M. Wainwright and his forces fought on until 6 May, when he surrendered to the Japanese with some 11,500 troops. Twenty-one Army nurses escaped from Corregidor before it fell to the Japanese. Under cover of darkness, 10 of the 21 Army nurses made the trip safely to Australia in a

PBY Catalina aircraft with approximately 25 other Army and Navy officers, crew members, and a few civilians. The other 11 Army nurses who escaped were evacuated by submarine.

6 May 1942 With the fall of Corregidor, 66 Army nurses remained in the Philippines as prisoners of war of the Japanese. The 54 Army nurses and a former Army nurse captured on Corregidor cared for American military patients there until 25 June 1942. In August, they were moved to the Santo Tomas Internment Camp for civilians. In September, they were joined by 10 Army nurses captured earlier on Mindanao. The first of two nurses captured at Baguio arrived a year later; the second nurse arrived from another prison camp on 4 February 1945, one day after their liberation. Although denied the privilege of caring for military patients at Santo Tomas, except for the few wounded during the liberation of the camp, they continued to care for the sick in a camp hospital under the able leadership of Capt. Maude C. Davison during their entire internment until relieved by Army nurses who arrived on 9 February 1945. The former Army nurse joined the Army Nurse Corps upon liberation, to make 67 who had been prisoners of the Japanese. On 18 February 1945, each of the Army nurse prisoners of war received the Bronze Star Medal and a promotion of one grade in ceremonies on Leyte before departing for the United States. The last nurse prisoner of war to remain on active duty with the Army Nurse Corps was Lt. Col. Hattie R. Brantley who retired on 1 February 1969.

30 Jun 1942 There were 12,475 Army nurses on active duty.

8 Nov 1942 Nurses landed in North Africa on the day of the invasion. They were members of the staff of the 48th Surgical Hospital, later reorganized as the 128th Evacuation Hospital.

22 Dec 1942 Public Law 828, 77th Congress, authorized the relative rank of Army Nurse Corps officers from second lieutenant through colonel. It also provided for pay and allowances approximately equal to those granted commissioned officers without dependents.

17 Jan 1943 The first nurse to receive an Air Medal for meritorious service was 2d Lt. Elsie Ott. Lieutenant Ott served as a nurse for five patients who were being evacuated from India to Washington, D.C. This was the first aerial evacuation flight in nursing history and the pioneer movement of transporting wounded soldiers by air over such a great distance (11,000 miles).

10 Feb 1943 Lt. Col. Florence A. Blanchfield became Acting Superintendent of the Army Nurse Corps due to the illness of Col. Julia O. Flikke, the incumbent Superintendent.

18 Feb 1943 The first class of Army Nurse Corps flight nurses was graduated by the School of Air Evacuation at Bowman Field, Kentucky. The honor graduate who received the first flight wings was 2d Lt. Geraldine Dishroom. Since there was no official insignia, Brig. Gen. David Grant, Air Surgeon and guest speaker, unpinned his insignia and pinned it to her uniform. Lieutenant Dishroom was with the first air evacuation team to land on OMAHA Beach after the Normandy invasion on 6 June 1944. Second Lt. Dorothy Shikoski, the second Army nurse to receive the Air Medal and the first woman to receive the award in the South Pacific, was decorated for displaying heroism following a crash landing at sea during a severe storm in the South Pacific theater.

30 Jun 1943 Col. Julia O. Flikke retired. Among her many contributions to Army nursing was the publication of her well-known book, *Nurses in Action*. Colonel Flikke was awarded an honorary degree as Doctor of Science by Wittenberg College in 1944.

30 Jun 1943 There were 36,607 Army nurses on active duty.

1 Jul 1943 Col. Florence A. Blanchfield became the seventh Superintendent of the Army Nurse Corps.

1 Jul 1943 Public Law 74, 78th Congress, established the United States Cadet Nurse Corps under the administration of the United States Public Health Service. After entering World War II, the United States was faced with a critical shortage of registered nurses nationwide. It was deemed more expedient and economical to strengthen the instructional staff and the facilities of existing civilian schools of nursing than to reinstitute the Army School of Nursing or start similar military hospital–based schools. Although the act was a defense measure, a precedent had been established—schools of nursing were given recognition as essential agencies in the protection of the nation's health. The total number who joined the Cadet Nurse Corps was 169,443. Of these, 124,065 were graduated from 1,125 of the nation's 1,300 schools of nursing. Senior Cadets served in federal or nonfederal hospitals or in other health agencies. By the end of the program, 17,475 Senior Cadets had served the federal government during the last six months of the program. The greatest number to graduate from a single school was 1,600 cadets from the University of Minnesota School of Nursing. Recruitment terminated on 15 October 1945, and the last cadets graduated in 1948. Federal funds provided for maintenance of the students the first 9 months, for tuition fees throughout the program, and for necessary expansion of educational and residential facilities. Cadets were provided free uniforms and a monthly stipend which ranged from $15 a month for the first 9 months as a pre-Cadet, $30 a month for the next 21 months as a Junior Cadet, and from $30 to $60 a month during the last 6 months as a

Senior Cadet. The Cadet Nurse Corps was composed of student trainees and was not a branch of the armed forces or of the civilian personnel force of the United States government. The training and experience did not constitute federal service, and therefore no veterans' benefits accrued. The Corps pledge was a statement of good intentions rather than a legal contract:

> "In consideration of the training, payments, and other benefits which are provided me as a member of the United States Cadet Nurse Corps, I agree that I will be available for military or other Federal, governmental, or essential civilian services for the duration of the present war."

The service of thousands of cadets is still on the record as an exceptionally valuable contribution to the United States during and following World War II.

19 Jul 1943 The first basic training centers, established to provide military orientation for Army nurses before their first duty assignment, were formally opened at Fort Devens, Massachusetts; Fort Sam Houston, Texas; and Camp McCoy, Wisconsin. The nurses were oriented to military nursing and other subjects, such as how to prepare for gas injuries, bivouac in the field, seek foxholes for cover, and purify water. In 1946, an eight-week orientation program for all newly commissioned officers was established at the Medical Field Service School, Brooke Army Medical Center, Fort Sam Houston, Texas. The nurses were oriented to military customs and other subjects, such as military medical, surgical, and psychiatric techniques; preventive medicine; supply and tactical information; and administration, including ward management.

8 Nov 1943 A plane carrying thirteen nurses and seventeen others crash landed in Albania. After more than six weeks behind German lines, courageous underground partisans helped all thirty Americans escape from Nazi-held territory.

27 Jan 1944 Army nurses waded ashore on Anzio beachhead in Italy five days after troop landings on 22 January 1944. Six Army nurses lost their lives during enemy bombing attacks in early February.

10 Jun 1944 Four days after the Normandy invasion, nurses of the 42d and 45th Field Hospitals and the 91st and 128th Evacuation Hospitals arrived in Normandy.

22 Jun 1944 Public Law 350, 78th Congress, granted Army nurses temporary commissions in the Army of the United States, with full pay and privileges of the grades from second lieutenant through colonel, for the duration of the emergency plus six months.

9 Jul 1944 Gardiner General Hospital, Chicago, Illinois, was dedicated to the memory of 2d Lt. Ruth M. Gardiner, the first Army nurse to be killed in a theater of operations during World War II. Lieutenant Gardiner, a flight nurse, was killed in a plane crash near Naknek, Alaska, on 27 July 1943, while on an air evacuation mission.

27 Sep 1944 Lt. Reba Z. Whittle of the 813th Medical Air Evacuation Transport Squadron became a prisoner of the Germans after the plane in which she was flying during an evacuation mission was shot down over Aachen.

6 Jan 1945 Secretary of War Henry L. Stimson recommended to President Franklin Delano Roosevelt that women nurses be drafted for the armed forces. The President proposed such legislation in his State of the Union Message. The House of Representatives passed a draft bill on 7 March 1945, but the Senate had not acted upon it before victory in Europe on 8 May 1945. The War Department notified the Senate on 24 May 1945 that legislation would not be necessary since an adequate number of nurses had volunteered to meet the anticipated needs of the war in the Pacific. No further action was taken.

28 Apr 1945 Six Army nurses and five Army medical officers were among some twenty-nine people killed when the hospital ship *Comfort*, loaded to capacity with wounded being evacuated from Okinawa, was attacked by a Japanese "suicide" plane.

8 May 1945 Victory in Europe. V–E Day was proclaimed on 8 May after the enemy forces surrendered on 7 May 1945. When the war in Europe ended there were more than fifty-two thousand Army nurses on active duty serving in 605 hospitals overseas and 454 hospitals in the United States.

Sep 1945 Following World War II, Army nurses became eligible for all veterans' benefits. Many former Army nurses attended colleges and universities in the postwar period under the Servicemen's Readjustment Act of 1944, commonly known as the "G.I. Bill of Rights."

2 Sep 1945 Victory in Japan. V–J Day was proclaimed on 2 September to celebrate Japan's acceptance of unconditional surrender terms on 14 August 1945. The Army Nurse Corps had reached a peak strength of more than fifty-seven thousand in August 1945.

In World War II, 201 Army nurses died, 16 as a result of enemy action. More than sixteen hundred nurses were decorated for meritorious service and bravery under fire. Decorations included the Distinguished Service Medal, Silver Star, Distinguished Flying Cross, Soldier's Medal, Bronze Star Medal, Air Medal, Legion of Merit, Army Commendation Medal, and the Purple Heart.

Five hospital ships and one general hospital used during the war were named after Army nurses who lost their lives in service during World War II Army nurses served at station and general hospitals throughout the continental United States. Overseas, they were assigned to hospital ships, flying ambulances, and hospital trains; to clearing stations; and to field, evacuation, and general hospitals. They served on beachheads from North Africa to Normandy and Anzio, in the Aleutians, Wales, Australia, Trinidad, India, Ireland, England, the Solomons, Newfoundland, Guam, Hawaii, New Guinea, New Caledonia, Puerto Rico, Panama, Iceland, Bataan, and Corregidor—wherever the American soldier could be found. They traveled in close support of the fighting men, endured relentless bombing and strafing on land, torpedoing at sea, and antiaircraft fire while evacuating the wounded by air. In Europe, during the major battle offensives, Army nurses assisted in developing the concept of recovery wards for immediate postoperative nursing care of patients. The flight nurses helped to establish the incredible record of only five deaths in flight per 100,000 patients transported.

Lt. Frances Y. Slanger, in her tent in Belgium, far from home in Roxbury, Massachusetts, was one of the Army nurses who signed a letter written to *Stars and Stripes*:

> "Sure we rough it. But compared to the way you men are taking it we can't complain, nor do we feel that bouquets are due us . . . it is to you we doff our helmets. To every G.I. wearing the American uniform—for you we have the greatest admiration and respect."

Seventeen days later, on 21 October 1944, Lieutenant Slanger died of wounds caused by the shelling of her tented hospital area. Through the same newspaper, hundreds of soldiers replied:

> "To all Army nurses overseas: We men were not given the choice of working in the battlefield or the home front. We cannot take any credit for being here. We are here because we have to be. You are here because you felt you were needed. So, when an injured man opens his eyes to see one of you . . . concerned with his welfare, he can't but be overcome by the very thought that you are doing it because you want to . . . you endure whatever hardships you must to be where you can do us the most good."

31 Dec 1945 There were 27,850 Army nurses on active duty.

1946 During the occupation of Japan, Maj. Grace E. Alt organized a Nursing Education Council in Japan. Army nurses offered refresher courses to nurses and to nurse instructors of Japanese schools of nursing. Major Alt also helped to train Japanese nurses for public health work during the postwar period.

15 Jun 1946 A 26-week course in psychiatric nursing was introduced at Brooke Army Medical Center, Fort Sam Houston, Texas. This course marked the beginning of Army-wide education in clinical nursing practice. Training in clinical nursing procedures had been conducted to meet the Army's needs during World War II, but this 26-week course included 230 hours of formal classroom instruction at the Medical Field Service School and 580 hours of practicum with clinical demonstration at Brooke General Hospital. Several Army nurses were also selected to attend a similar course in psychiatric nursing at the St. Elizabeth Hospital, Washington, D.C.

30 Sep 1946 A year after the end of World War II, approximately eighty-five hundred nurses remained in the Army Nurse Corps.

16 Apr 1947 Public Law 36, 80th Congress, established the Army Nurse Corps in the Medical Department of the Regular Army and authorized a strength of not less than 2,558 nurses. The Army-Navy Nurse Act of 1947 also provided permanent commissioned officer status for members of the Army Nurse Corps in the grades of second lieutenant through lieutenant colonel, and for the Chief of the Army Nurse Corps to serve in the temporary grade of colonel. The act also established the Army Nurse Corps Section of the Officers' Reserve Corps.

Army nurses on active duty who held Regular relative rank in the Army Nurse Corps as well as a temporary commission were appointed in an appropriate permanent grade but continued to serve in their temporary grade if the latter was higher. Reserve nurses, on either active or inactive status, who met the qualifications for Regular Army appointment were given the opportunity to apply. A total of 894 Army Nurse Corps officers were integrated into the Regular Army.

11 Jun 1947 Lt. Col. Ida W. Danielson was awarded the Florence Nightingale Medal by the International Red Cross in recognition of her work as Director of Nurses, European Theater of Operations, from February 1944 through October 1945.

19 Jun 1947 Col. Florence A. Blanchfield, Chief of the Army Nurse Corps, was given United States Army serial number N–1 and commissioned in the permanent grade of lieutenant colonel in the Regular Army. She thus became the first woman to hold a permanent commission in the United States Army. As Chief of the Army Nurse Corps, she continued to serve in the temporary grade of colonel.

1 Jul 1947 A 56-week course in anesthesiology for nurses was started at four hospitals: Brooke General Hospital, Fort Sam Houston, Texas; Fitzsimons General Hospital, Denver, Colorado; Letterman General Hospital, San Francisco, California; and Walter Reed General Hospital, Washington, D.C. Forty weeks of this 56-week course were spent in an Army hospital and eight weeks in an approved civilian hospital for clinical experience with types of anesthesia not commonly used in Army hospitals. The first course included 359 hours of lecture, not less than 375 cases, and not less than 375 hours of actual administration of anesthesia. Upon graduation, the nurse was qualified to take the examination prepared by the American Association of Nurse Anesthetists. Certification was granted upon successful completion of the examination.

21 Jul 1947 The first course in operating room technique and management for nurses (later changed to operating room nursing and administration) to prepare for Army certification as an operating room specialist was introduced at two hospitals: Letterman General Hospital, San Francisco, California, and Walter Reed General Hospital, Washington, D.C. The course at Walter Reed was affiliated with the School of Nursing, The Catholic University of America, Washington, D.C. This 24-week course included 155 hours of classroom instruction and 668 hours of supervised clinical practice.

30 Sep 1947 Col. Florence A. Blanchfield, Chief of the Army Nurse Corps, retired after more than twenty-nine years of active service. The Army awarded her the Distinguished Service Medal on 14 June 1945 for her leadership of the Corps during World War II. Colonel Blanchfield received many honors including the Florence Nightingale Medal, awarded by the International Red Cross on 12 May 1951, and the Distinguished Service Medal from her native state of West Virginia on 19 July 1963.

1 Oct 1947 Col. Mary G. Phillips became the eighth Chief of the Army Nurse Corps. Colonel Phillips was the first graduate of the Army School of Nursing to serve as Chief of the Corps.

10 Nov 1947 For the first time, Army nurses attended the course in hospital administration at the Army Medical Field Service School. A graduate-level program was started in 1951. Through an affiliation with Baylor University, the first master of hospital administration degrees were awarded to Army Medical Department officers in 1953. The program has since become the U.S. Army–Baylor University graduate program in Health Care Administration. The two-year program includes a didactic year at the Academy of Health Sciences, U.S. Army, Fort Sam Houston, Texas, followed by a residency year, under the direction of an approved preceptor, at an Army hospital. Upon successful completion of the program, a master of hospital administration degree is conferred by Baylor University, Waco, Texas.

31 Dec 1947 Army Nurse Corps strength was 4,859: Regular Army, 925; reserve officers on active duty, 3,934.

9 Jun 1948 The first civilian nursing leaders were appointed as consultants to the Surgeon General for matters pertaining to Army nursing. They were: Katherine Densford (later Mrs. Dreves), Director, School of Nursing, University of Minnesota; Agnes Gelinas, Chairman, Department of Nursing, Skidmore College; Ella Best, Executive Secretary of the American Nurses' Association (ANA); and Lulu St. Clair Blaine, Executive Secretary, Michigan Nursing Center Association.

28 Aug 1948 The five Army Nurse Corps officers to attend the first Medical Department Officers Advanced Course, Medical Field Service School, were Lt. Col. Ruby F. Bryant, Lt. Col. Pauline Kirby, Maj. Inez Haynes, Maj. Margaret Harper, and Capt. Harriet A. Dawley (Wells). Lieutenant Colonel Bryant, Major Haynes, and Major Harper later became Chiefs of the Army Nurse Corps. Captain Dawley (Wells) later became Assistant Chief of the Corps. In 1956, Lieutenant Colonel Kirby was promoted to the temporary grade of colonel. She was one of the first two Army Nurse Corps officers, other than the Chief of the Corps, to serve in the temporary grade of colonel.

1949 Reserve nurses on active or inactive duty were authorized and encouraged to take extension courses, on their own time, in technical or administrative procedures. Reserve nurses not on active duty could request assignment for training purposes to reserve units near their homes to maintain proficiency in nursing practice related to the latest advances in military medicine.

1 Feb 1949 The first Army Health Nurse Program was established at Fort Devens, Massachusetts, to provide public health nursing services to the military community.

Jul 1949 The role of the Nursing Methods Analyst in Army hospitals began to evolve after Executive Order 10072 was issued in July 1949. Following World War II, the Hoover Commission was appointed to study the organization and administration of the various federal agencies. In its report to Congress, the commission outlined the need for all agencies to study their efficiency and economy of operation. By Executive Order 10072, the President of the United States directed all departmental and agency heads to give attention to the organization and administration of their departments.

In October 1949, Congress passed Public Law 429. This law established in all the federal agencies, including the Department of Defense, the legal basis for a comprehensive and continuing program of management improvement.

The Bureau of the Budget was charged with the responsibility of coordinating the program. The Secretary of the Army established the management program at the Department of the Army level.

In the Office of the Surgeon General, the program was developed in the Medical Plans and Operations Division and was called the Management Research and Planning Branch. As early as 1946, a management research group had already been appointed in the Office of the Surgeon General and assigned to do research in the field of hospital operations.

In 1949, Valley Forge General Hospital was selected as the Army hospital where pilot projects to improve hospital organization and administration would be conducted. Lt. Col. Daisy M. McCommons was Chief Nurse. (In 1950, she was assigned to the Management Research and Planning Branch, Office of the Surgeon General.) Lt. Col. Arthur Stout, MSC, was Chief of the Management Office at Valley Forge Hospital. The first Army nurses assigned to the hospital management program were Capt. Robena Anderson and 1st Lt. Eileen L. McCarthy. They were joined a few months later by Capt. Ann Witczak.

The objective of the first survey was to determine standards of staffing for nursing service in Army hospitals through use of the nursing team. The initial study, formally conducted from January to June 1950, was interrupted because the Secretary of Defense ordered the hospital closed by 30 June 1950 as an economy measure. The hospital was reopened during the Korean War, and management nurses were assigned to resume management studies at Valley Forge and to continue at other Army hospitals.

In 1950, the management office in Army hospitals was established as a fact-finding, planning, advisory, and control agency, on the authority of Surgeon General's Office Circular 119 and SR 40–610–5. The management nurse was included in the management office. The title changed variously until 1959 from Management Nurse, to Nursing Management Nurse, to Nursing Methods Analyst (NMA).

By mid-1975, nursing methods analysts were assigned to Army medical centers and general hospitals throughout the Health Services Command. For more than twenty-five years, nursing methods analysts have been a part of the Army medical team charged with the responsibility for patient care planning, manpower utilization, facilities planning, and supplies and equipment requirements. They have made many lasting contributions to the Army Medical Department. For example, centralization of the food service in Army hospitals came into being as a result of one of the utilization studies conducted by nursing methods analysts. Another significant contribution, resulting from a study conducted from 1951 to 1955 in eight Army hospitals, was "categorization of patients according to nursing care needs"—a standard for determining staffing requirements for nursing personnel in Army hospitals and a forerunner of the progressive patient care concept of intensive, moderate, minimal, and supportive care.

1 Jul 1949 The Air Force Nurse Corps was established. A total of 1,199 Army nurses on active duty (307 regular and 892 reserve officers) transferred from the Army to the Air Force and formed the nucleus of its Nurse Corps.

17 Oct 1949 A 48-week pilot course of instruction for enlisted personnel on the practical nurse level was started at the Army Medical Center, Washington, D.C. (later renamed the Walter Reed Army Medical Center). The program was similar to the one-year program for practical nurses at the University of Minnesota. The Army program was the forerunner of the Medical Technician Procedure Advanced Course. The director and faculty members were Army Nurse Corps officers. Additional schools, under the direction of Army Nurse Corps officers, were established as required to meet patient care needs of the Army Medical Service. The course was retitled the Medical Specialist (Advanced) Course and, later, the Clinical Specialist Course.

25 Jun 1950 Capt. Viola B. McConnell was the only Army nurse on duty in Korea at the start of hostilities. Assigned to the United States Military Advisory Group to the Republic of Korea, Captain McConnell escorted nearly seven hundred American evacuees, mostly women and children, from besieged Seoul to Japan aboard the Norwegian freighter *Rheinhold*, a ship which normally had accommodations for only twelve passengers. The crew members gave up their quarters for the infants and children. Captain McConnell assessed priorities for care of the evacuees and worked with a medical team organized from the passengers, including one United Nations nurse, one Army wife (a registered nurse), six missionary nurses, and one medical missionary (a woman doctor described by Captain McConnell as "magnificent—and she worked long hours. . . we will be ever grateful to her for her assistance"). Captain McConnell requested assignment back to Korea from Japan. She later returned to Taejon to aid in the care and evacuation of the wounded men of the 24th Division. Captain McConnell was awarded the Bronze Star Medal for her heroic performance of duty in assisting with the evacuation of Americans from Seoul and, later, the Oak Leaf Cluster to the Bronze Star Medal for her outstanding service in Korea.

27 Jun 1950 President Harry S. Truman ordered U.S. air and naval forces into the Republic of Korea (South Korea).

1 Jul 1950 The first U.S. Army combat units landed in Korea after U.S. ground forces were ordered into the fighting in South Korea on 30 June 1950.

5 Jul 1950 Fifty-seven Army nurses arrived in Pusan, Korea. They helped set up a hospital and were caring for patients by the following day. Two days later, on 8 July 1950, twelve Army nurses moved forward with a mobile Army surgical hospital (MASH) to Taejon on the perimeter. By August, more than one hundred Army nurses were on duty in South Korea in support of United Nations troops. During the first year of the Korean conflict, the strength of the Army Nurse Corps increased from 3,460 on 15 July 1950 to 5,397 in July 1951.

Throughout the ground fighting until 1951, and during the prolonged peace negotiations that lasted until 27 July 1953, approximately 540 Army Nurse Corps officers served throughout the Korean peninsula. They served in twenty-five medical treatment facilities, such as mobile Army surgical hospitals; evacuation, field, and station hospitals; and hospital trains.

Army nurses supported combat troops during the amphibious attack and landing on Inchon in western Korea, well behind the Pusan beachhead line; the advance across the 38th Parallel toward North Korea in the west; the amphibious landing on the east coast of Korea pushing toward the Yalu River, the northern boundary of Korea; and the disastrous defeat when they were forced to retreat well below the 38th Parallel. Their support continued as allied forces pushed back the Chinese, regaining practically all of South Korea plus a few hundred square miles north of the parallel. Maj. Gen. Edgar Erskine Hume, Surgeon, United Nations Command and Far East Command, paid tribute to Army nurses in Korea:

> "Members of the Army Nurse Corps have all distinguished themselves by their devotion to duty, their utter disregard of working hours, and their willingness to do anything that needs to be done at any time. They have displayed courage, stamina and determination. They have completed every task with which they have been confronted in a superior manner."

No Army nurse was killed due to enemy action in Korea, but the story of the Army Nurse Corps in the Korean War would not be complete without mention of the tragic and untimely death of Maj. Genevieve Smith of Epworth, Iowa. Major Smith, a veteran of World War II, was among the victims of a C–47 crash while en route to her duty assignment as Chief Nurse in Korea.

Aug 1950 The Army Nurse Corps was exempted from the Army-wide requirement that all commissioned officers hold or achieve a baccalaureate degree. The majority of registered nurses nationwide were graduates of a three-year hospital (diploma) program. By August 1950, only two years had passed since the last of 124,065 Cadet Nurse Corps participants had graduated.

Relatively few degree-completion programs were available for diploma graduates. Nonetheless, the goal set in 1950 was for Army Nurse Corps officers to complete an accredited program leading to an undergraduate degree, preferably in nursing.

5 Sep 1950 The first course in nursing administration, which later became the Military Nursing Advanced Course, was established at the U.S. Army Medical Field Service School, Fort Sam Houston, Texas. The twenty-week course included principles of nursing administration, current trends in nursing, principles of supervision and teaching, hospital organization and functions, personnel administration, psychology of leadership, and orientation to all departments of an Army hospital.

1951 Maj. Elizabeth Pagels became the first Army Health Nurse to be assigned to the Preventive Medicine Division, Professional Service Directorate, Office of the Surgeon General, to assist with issues related to the practice of Army health nursing.

2 Feb 1951 The fiftieth anniversary of the Army Nurse Corps was observed throughout the world.

26 Jun 1951 The American Red Cross awarded the cherished Florence Nightingale Medal to Col. Florence A. Blanchfield (Ret.), seventh Superintendent of the Army Nurse Corps, "for exceptional service on behalf of humanity rendered through the Red Cross."

29 Jun 1951 Department of Defense (DOD) Directive 750.04–1 (renumbered 1125.1) established a definitive policy on the utilization of registered nurses in the military services. Registered nurses were to be relieved of custodial and housekeeping duties and clerical, food service, and other nonnursing functions in patient care areas. The DOD directive also instructed the various military medical services to institute programs to train and utilize more practical nurses and other nonprofessional nursing service personnel in staffing for patient care.

Even before the Department of Defense policy was established, plans were being developed and projects had been initiated under the aegis of management improvement which would work toward solving the problems of defining and staffing the nursing service. The studies ultimately resulted in the reorganization of nursing service in Army hospitals. Duties and functions of registered nurses were defined. A 48-week pilot course of instruction for enlisted personnel on the practical nurse level had already been instituted in 1949. On-the-job training programs were developed for both professional and nonprofessional nursing personnel. As a result of concerted efforts to comply with the DOD directive, Army Nurse Corps officers were authorized, after 8 September 1953, technical control of enlisted personnel assigned to nursing service.

11 Aug 1951 The Defense Advisory Committee on Women in the Services (DACOWITS) was established by the Secretary of Defense to interpret to the public the role of women in the services and to promote acceptance of military service as a career for women.

30 Sep 1951 Col. Mary G. Phillips retired. Colonel Phillips was the first Chief of the Army Nurse Corps to complete the statutory four-year appointment as Chief of the Corps. Among the honors received by Colonel Phillips was the Legion of Merit on 23 October 1945 for her outstanding service as First Assistant to the Superintendent, Army Nurse Corps.

1 Oct 1951 Col. Ruby F. Bryant became the ninth Chief of the Army Nurse Corps. Colonel Bryant was the second graduate of the Army School of Nursing to serve as Chief of the Corps.

Jun 1952 A career guidance program for Army Nurse Corps officers was established in the Office of the Surgeon General. Capt. Harriet H. Werley was assigned as the first career guidance counselor.

30 Dec 1953 The Registered Nurse Student Program (RNSP) was established to recruit registered nurses for the Army Nurse Corps. The program provided financial assistance, pay, and allowances of grade in which commissioned to registered nurses in their final year of study for a bachelor's or master's degree in a field of nursing. Upon graduation, they were obligated to serve as reserve officers on active duty for two years. Grade in which commissioned, from second lieutenant through captain, depended on qualifications by education and experience. Authorization for men to apply for the program was approved on 20 November 1962.

13 Feb 1954 The first two professional postgraduate short courses were established for nurses: one in operating room nursing at Walter Reed Army Medical Center, Washington, D.C.; and one in nursing service administration at Brooke Army Medical Center, Fort Sam Houston, Texas.

31 Mar 1954 A Medical Training Center was established at Brooke Army Medical Center, Fort Sam Houston, Texas, to replace the training center for enlisted personnel of the Army Medical Service at Camp Pickett, Virginia, which was scheduled for closing in June 1954. Army nurses continued to serve on the faculty as full-time instructors.

14 Jan 1955 The Stimson Library at the U.S. Army Medical Field Service School, Brooke Army Medical Center, Fort Sam Houston, Texas, was dedicated to the memory of Col. Julia C. Stimson, fifth Superintendent of the Army Nurse Corps. In January 1973, the Stimson Library was moved from the former Medical Field Service School to the new Academy of Health Sciences, U.S. Army, Fort Sam Houston, Texas.

Feb 1955 A 22-week course in obstetrical nursing was started at Walter Reed General Hospital, Washington, D.C. The course was transferred to William Beaumont General Hospital, El Paso, Texas, in March 1959. It was expanded to include the concept of child health and retitled Maternal and Child Health Nursing. This course was discontinued in 1971.

14 Feb 1955 Closed-circuit color television was used for the first time in Army nursing instruction when surgical procedures in the operating room at Walter Reed General Hospital, Washington, D.C., were transmitted to the Military Operating Room Workshop at the Army Medical Service Graduate School (later renamed the Walter Reed Army Institute of Research), Walter Reed Army Medical Center, Washington, D.C.

12 May 1955 Thompson Hall was dedicated at Letterman General Hospital, San Francisco, California, in memory of Capt. Dora E. Thompson, fourth Superintendent of the Army Nurse Corps. Miss Thompson had served as Chief Nurse at Letterman at the time of the 1906 earthquake and fire and, again, before her retirement in 1942.

15 Jun 1955 Lt. Col. Ruby G. Bradley was awarded the Florence Nightingale Medal by the International Red Cross for outstanding service when she was a prisoner of war of the Japanese during World War II and for her service in Korea. When she retired on 31 March 1963, Colonel Bradley received the third Oak Leaf Cluster to the Legion of Merit. She held the distinction of being the most decorated woman in the history of the United States Army. On 1 June 1964, Colonel Bradley was awarded an honorary degree as Doctor of Science by the University of West Virginia.

9 Aug 1955 Public Law 294, 84th Congress, introduced by Mrs. Frances P. Bolton, Representative from Ohio, and signed by President Dwight D. Eisenhower, authorized commissions for male nurses in the U.S. Army Reserve for assignment to the Army Nurse Corps Branch. Mrs. Bolton had earlier introduced H.R. 911 on 4 January 1951 in an attempt to provide for the appointment of men as nurses in the Army, the Navy, and the Air Force.

19 Aug 1955 Capt. Ruth Dickson was awarded the Associate Royal Red Cross by Her Britannic Majesty's government. The decoration, comparable to the

American Distinguished Service Cross, was awarded to Captain Dickson for her service to British Commonwealth Forces in Korea while she served as Chief Nurse of the 8055th Mobile Army Surgical Hospital (MASH).

30 Sep 1955 Col. Ruby F. Bryant, upon completion of the statutory four-year term as Chief of the Army Nurse Corps, reverted, by law, to her permanent grade of lieutenant colonel (until after Public Law 85–155 was passed by Congress on 13 August 1957) and was assigned as Chief, Nursing Service, Medical Division, Europe. She later served as Director, Nursing Activities, Brooke Army Medical Center, Fort Sam Houston, Texas, until she retired on 30 June 1961. Colonel Bryant was the recipient of many honors, including the Legion of Merit awarded upon retirement. She also received an honorary Doctor of Law degree from the Medical College of Virginia, Richmond, Virginia, on 31 May 1955.

1 Oct 1955 Col. Inez Haynes became the tenth Chief of the Army Nurse Corps.

6 Oct 1955 Edward L.T. Lyon, a nurse anesthetist from Kings Park, New York, was commissioned a second lieutenant in the Army Nurse Corps Reserve and entered active duty on 10 October 1955. Lieutenant Lyon was the first man to receive a commission in the Army Nurse Corps.

18 Apr 1956 The Army Student Nurse Program (ASNP) was designed to help solve the acute shortage of nurses in the Army. The ASNP provided financial assistance, pay, and allowances of private, first class (E–3), to nursing students, both men and women, at the end of their second year in either a three- or four-year program, and at the end of their third year in a five-year program. The schools of nursing were approved by the Department of the Army and accredited by the National League for Nursing. Upon successful completion of the ASNP and state licensure, the participant was commissioned a second lieutenant in the U.S. Army Reserve and obligated to serve on active duty for two or three years, depending on the length of time in the nursing program.

In December 1960, the Army Student Nurse Program was revised to authorize the participant, enrolled in the last two years of a four-year degree-granting school of nursing, to be commissioned six months before graduation and to receive full pay and allowances of the grade held during the last six months of student status. The 1960 revision also permitted payment of tuition, books, and incidental fees. In November 1961, the ASNP was opened to graduates of a hospital school of nursing (diploma) program to complete their baccalaureate degree if they could graduate within twenty-four months.

29 Apr 1956 Three Army nurses, Maj. Frances K. Smith, her sister, Maj. Helen D. Smith, and Maj. Jane Becker, were placed on temporary duty assignment with the United States Military Assistance Advisory Group (MAAG) in Saigon, Vietnam. The First Indochina War between France and the Vietnamese Communists had ended just two years earlier with the Geneva Accords of 1954. Their primary missions were to train South Vietnamese nurses in nursing care procedures and to provide patient care to MAAG personnel.

26 Jul 1956 The Evangeline G. Bovard Award was established by Col. Robert Skelton, Medical Corps, in memory of his wife, who had served as an Army nurse from 1912 to 1917 and died at Letterman General Hospital in 1955. Selection of the Army Nurse Corps officer(s) for this award, presented annually at Letterman, is based on demonstration of the highest degree of professional competence and outstanding performance of duty. Capt. Lenora B. Weirick was the first recipient on 14 January 1958; see Appendix D.)

Nov 1956 During the Hungarian uprising in Europe, Army Nurse Corps officers served with Army Medical Service units in Operation MERCY. They cared for refugees both in Europe and at Camp Kilmer, New Jersey.

7 Nov 1956 Lt. Cols. Pauline Kirby and Agnes A. Maley were promoted to the temporary grade of colonel in the Army of the United States. They were the first two Army Nurse Corps officers, other than the Chief of the Corps, to serve in the temporary grade of colonel, AUS.

3 Dec 1956 The first three male nurses reported to Fort Campbell, Kentucky, for airborne training.

25 Feb 1957 A Department of Nursing was established at the Walter Reed Army Institute of Research, Walter Reed Army Medical Center, Washington, D.C., with the primary mission of providing education and conducting research in clinical nursing practice. Maj. Harriet H. Werley, M.S. in nursing administration from Teachers College, Columbia University, New York, became its first Chief. The first nursing studies included those on decubitus ulcer care, oral hygiene, body temperature readings, and use of a plastic isolator for operating in a sterile environment.

Mar 1957 Capt. Margaret A. Ewen was the first Army Nurse Corps officer to serve in the Office of the Special Assistant to the Surgeon General for Reserve Affairs. At the request of the Office of the Surgeon General, Captain Ewen entered on active duty from U.S. Army Reserve status. Before reporting for active duty, Captain Ewen had been an assistant professor of nursing, School of Nursing, University of Pennsylvania.

5 Mar 1957 Davison Hall, a residence for women officers at Brooke Army Medical Center, Fort Sam Houston, Texas, was dedicated in honor of Maj.

Maude C. Davison. She had served in the Army of Occupation in Germany, World War I, and was Chief Nurse, Philippine Department, and Chief Nurse, U.S. Army Forces in the Philippines, when the United States entered World War II. After being taken prisoner of war by the Japanese on 7 May 1942, Captain Davison was Chief Nurse in charge of the nursing staff at the Santo Tomas Internment Camp, Philippine Islands, until she was relieved by Army nurses who arrived on 9 February 1945. Major Davison retired on 31 January 1946.

May 1957 Seven Army nurses participated in Operation PLUMBBOB, biochemical research conducted in conjunction with nuclear detonation testing at Mercury, Nevada. They helped evaluate the effects of atomic blast on swine. Capt. Ethylene Hughes was instrumental in planning and implementing nursing activities in support of this six-month project.

3 Jun 1957 Second Lt. Dclores M. Gleich, an honor graduate of South Dakota State College at Brookings, South Dakota, and 2d Lt. Audrey A. Johnson, a graduate of Augustana College at Sioux Falls, South Dakota, were the first two participants of the Army Student Nurse Program to receive commissions in the Army Nurse Corps Reserve and report for a two-year tour of active duty.

13 Aug 1957 Career opportunities for Regular Army nurses were improved by the enactment of Public Law 85–155, 85th Congress, signed by President Dwight D. Eisenhower. The law changed the age and grade provisions for appointment in the Regular Army; provided for 5 colonels and 107 lieutenant colonels; eliminated the restriction on the number authorized to serve in the grade of major; established a separate list for promotion for ANC officers; retained mandatory retirement at age sixty; provided retirement pay equal to all other officers in the Regular Army; and authorized retirement in a grade equal to the highest temporary grade held for six months. It also authorized a strength of 2,500 for the Regular Army Nurse Corps. By 29 February 1960, approximately 700 nurses had been promoted to the grade of major and more than 250 were on the recommended list for temporary promotion to major.

13 Sep 1957 Maj. Kathleen W. Phillips, who won national recognition in the field of audiovisual education, was assigned as Consultant, Nursing Audio-Visual Education, Medical Illustration Service, at the Armed Forces Institute of Pathology, Washington, D.C.

4 Mar 1958 Col. Inez Haynes, Chief of the Army Nurse Corps, and Lt. Cols. Ruby F. Bryant and Ruby G. Bradley were promoted to the grade of colonel in the Regular Army. They were the first women officers to hold the Regular Army permanent grade of colonel.

27 Jun 1958 The courses in operating room nursing and administration at Letterman General Hospital, San Francisco, California, and Walter Reed General Hospital, Washington, D C , were discontinued A 22-week course in basic operating room nursing was started at two hospitals. Letterman General Hospital, San Francisco, and the United States Army Hospital, Fort Benning, Georgia

Jul 1958 The Army Nurse Corps joined with the National League for Nursing (NLN) in the Disaster Nursing Project financed by the Federal Civil Defense Administration. Four Army Nurse Corps officers, three on active duty and one U.S. Army Reserve officer not on active duty, were assigned to develop courses on disaster nursing to be introduced in the curriculum at civilian schools of nursing Lt. Col. Ida Graham Price served at Teachers College, Columbia University; Capt. Drusilla Poole at the University of Minnesota; Capt. Virginia Farrell at Massachusetts General Hospital; and Maj. Grace Davidson, ANC, USAR, remained working with Skidmore College. Although the NLN project was a five-year endeavor, the Army Nurse Corps officers served for one year assigned to the Department of Nursing, Walter Reed Army Institute of Research, with duty station at the respective civilian schools of nursing.

26 Jul 1958 During the Lebanon crisis (July–October), Army Nurse Corps officers were assigned on the staffs of the 58th Evacuation Hospital and the 4th Surgical Hospital which supported over ten thousand American troops in Lebanon. Twenty-one Army nurses—nineteen women and two men—were with the first contingent of the 400-bed 58th Evacuation Hospital airlift from the Seventh U. S. Army, USAREUR (Germany), to the hospital site near Beirut.

Oct 1958 For the first time, Army Nurse Corps officers were assigned to airborne divisions. Three men were assigned to each of the two medical units. In addition to their duties as Army Nurse Corps officers, the men had to be jump qualified

11 Jan 1959 Mary M. Roberts, R.N., writer, editor, historian, and a member of the Army Nurse Corps in World War I, died at the age of 82. Miss Roberts was Editor Emeritus of the *American Journal of Nursing* and won acclaim as the author of "American Nursing· History and Interpretation," and "The Army Nurse Corps, Yesterday and Today." The latter publication was distributed by the U.S. Army to libraries and schools of nursing in the United States.

22 Jul 1959 Criteria for determining the initial grade of officers for appointment in the Army Nurse Corps were revised to include credit for educational preparation beyond the basic nursing education program. Additional credit for educational preparation was authorized on 2 May 1960.

31 Aug 1959 Col. Inez Haynes, Chief of the Army Nurse Corps, retired and accepted the position of General Director of the National League for Nursing. Colonel Haynes was the recipient of many awards, including the Legion of Merit and University of Minnesota's Outstanding Achievement Award.

1 Sep 1959 Col. Margaret Harper became the eleventh Chief of the Army Nurse Corps.

28 Sep 1959 A 37-week course in advanced operating room nursing was introduced at Walter Reed General Hospital.

28 Jan 1960 Lt. Col. Edythe Turner was promoted to temporary colonel in the United States Army Reserve. Colonel Turner thus became the first career Army Reserve nurse to serve in the grade of colonel.

26 May 1960 Army nurses served in the hospitals which were airlifted to Chile to aid the victims of a severe earthquake and tidal wave. The two hospitals which participated in relief operations during May and June were the 7th Field, with thirty nurses, from Fort Belvoir, Virginia, and the 15th Field, with thirty nurses, from Fort Bragg, North Carolina.

2 Jun 1960 Army Regulations No. 611–103 provided the criteria for awarding letter or digit prefixes for classifying Army Nurse Corps officers according to military occupational specialty (MOS). The purpose of the classification was to conserve available skills of highly prepared nurses, improve the balance in clinical specialty areas, reflect the need for advanced preparation in the clinical specialty areas, aid in the development of career patterns, help in the construction of tables of distribution and organization, improve the procedures for requisition and assignment of personnel, and more accurately report and inventory nurses by specialty and authorized strength by position title. By 5 September 1961, the review and reclassification of more than three thousand Army Nurse Corps officers had been completed.

29 Jun 1960 Army Regulations No. 350–200 regarding long-term civilian schooling prescribed that the requirement for a baccalaureate degree be completed before age thirty-two and a master's degree before age thirty-seven.

1 Jul 1960 An award sponsored by the Association of the United States Army was established to be given to the outstanding student of each Army Nurse Corps Officers Basic Course, U.S. Army Medical Field Service School, Brooke Army Medical Center, Fort Sam Houston, Texas. Capt. Delores H. Randall was the first recipient on 9 December 1960.

13 Jul 1960 Prior active duty in the U S. Army Reserve was eliminated as a prerequisite for a commission as an Army Nurse Corps officer in the Regular Army. The direct commission of civilian nurses was authorized, and the need for certain candidates to appear before the Regular Army Selection Board was deleted from Army regulations

17 Aug 1960 The Army Nurse Corps Medal Fund was established through funds voluntarily contributed by active duty and retired Army nurses. The funds provided for a medal to be awarded to the graduate of each Military Nursing Advanced Course at the U.S. Army Medical Field Service School who best exemplified the ideal military nurse. The course was later retitled the Army Nurse Corps Officers Career Course. Capt. Angeline Hennek received the first medal on 9 June 1961. (See Appendix H.)

Dec 1960 The Degree Completion Program authorized up to twelve calendar months for completion of requirements for a bachelor's degree and six months for a master's degree. Regular Army and career reserve officers were eligible for the program.

1 Jul 1961 A twelve-month Army health nurse training program was established to prepare Army Nurse Corps officers to assume the responsibilities for the health nurse program at military posts and stations. Opportunities for graduate study were made available to experienced career Army health nurses.

11 Jul 1961 Army nurses participated in relief operations following the crash of United Airlines Flight 759 near Denver, Colorado. The 249th General Hospital was dispatched to the crash scene Fitzsimons General Hospital provided inpatient hospitalization.

14 Jul 1961 Appointment criteria for commissioning as an Army Nurse Corps officer required the applicant to be a graduate of a school of nursing whose curriculum was not less than thirty months, exclusive of vacation time.

26 Aug 1961 The Berlin Wall was built in Berlin, Germany, creating a war scare. Army nurses were among the medical personnel of twenty-two United States Army Reserve and National Guard units ordered to active duty on 1 October 1961 to increase Army strength during a period of international tension.

28 Aug 1961 The first forty-week course in military nursing practice and research was conducted at the Walter Reed Army Institute of Research, Walter Reed Army Medical Center, Washington, D.C.

5 Sep 1961 The Directors of the Army Distaff Foundation determined that retired Army Nurse Corps officers were eligible for residence at the newly constructed Distaff Hall on the same basis as Army widows.

15 Nov 1961 To increase the strength of the Army Nurse Corps during an Army-wide buildup, commissioning criteria were changed to allow reserve officers who had not passed their fortieth birthday and were majors or below to apply for one year of active duty. On 28 November 1961, applicants for commissions, including those in the Army Student Nurse Program and civilian registered nurses, could apply in advance to attend one of five courses in a clinical area: anesthesiology for nurses (18 months), Army health nursing (12 months), maternal and child health (5 months), operating room (5 months), or psychiatric nursing (4 months).

28 Nov 1961 Lt. Col. Ruth P. Satterfield, Director of the Anesthesiology Course for Nurses at Walter Reed General Hospital, became the first Army nurse not assigned to the Office of the Surgeon General to serve as a consultant to the Surgeon General when she assumed the additional duty of consultant in anesthesiology nursing.

Jan 1962 Six-month formal supervised clinical training programs in psychiatric nursing were established to qualify nurses for the MOS 3437, Neuropsychiatric Nursing, at Brooke General Hospital, Fort Sam Houston, Texas; Fitzsimons General Hospital, Denver, Colorado; Letterman General Hospital, San Francisco, California; and Valley Forge General Hospital, Phoenixville, Pennsylvania.

9 Jan 1962 Army Regulations No. 611–103 granted the military General Educational Development (GED) equivalent of two years at college level to Army Nurse Corps officers who were graduates of a hospital (diploma) school of nursing.

16 Jan 1962 The responsibility for Army nurse recruitment programs was transferred from the Office of the Surgeon General to the Deputy Chief of Staff for Personnel, Department of the Army. Army nurses were assigned to the U.S. Army Recruiting Service, Fort Monroe, Virginia. Army Nurse Corps counselors, with the support of the Recruiting Service, including assistance from enlisted recruiters, coordinated and implemented a program on a nationwide basis to interpret the need and opportunities for nurses in the Army.

Mar 1962 The first contingent of ten Army nurses arrived in the Republic of Vietnam. They were assigned to the 8th Field Hospital, Nha Trang. The hospital became operational on 18 April 1962. Its mission during the three years before the buildup of American forces in 1965 was to support U.S. Army personnel in South Vietnam. Five Army nurses were later assigned to a dispensary which opened in 1964 at Soc Trang before the 3d Field Hospital arrived in Saigon in April 1965.

17 May 1962 Eleven Army nurses were the first to be assigned to the staff of the 31st Field Hospital, Korat, Thailand.

21 May 1962 Maj. Lawrence W. Scheffner was the first man in the Army Nurse Corps to be assigned to the Office of the Surgeon General. Major Scheffner served in the Army Nurse Corps Assignment Branch of the Personnel and Training Directorate.

Jul 1962 The course in Anesthesiology for Nurses was revised and extended from twelve to eighteen months. The fifth program was started at William Beaumont General Hospital, El Paso, Texas, in October 1962. A year later, the sixth was started at Madigan General Hospital, Tacoma, Washington. The seventh was started at Tripler Army Medical Center, Hawaii, on 1 November 1965.

4 Sep 1962 Army nurses served in the hospital unit which was airlifted to Iran to aid the victims of a disastrous earthquake on 1 September 1962 which claimed more than ten thousand lives. The 8th Evacuation Hospital dispatched a 120-bed unit, with twenty-one nurses, from the Seventh U.S. Army, USAREUR (Germany), to participate in relief operations from 4–23 September.

Oct 1962 Cuban Missile Crisis (October–December). Army nurses were dispatched with medical teams needed to participate in medical support operations worldwide during a period of international tension.

6 Nov 1962 Army Regulations No. 611–103 required the annual review and confirmation of an Army Nurse Corps officer's competence in a clinical specialty when it authorized the award of a specialty letter or digit prefix to the military occupational specialty. Use of the letter or digit prefix designated degrees of proficiency in terms of formal education and training, years of experience, and competency in a clinical specialty. It was recognized that grade and prefix would not necessarily parallel each other. The letter "A" prefix to the MOS is awarded only to those individuals in the Army Medical Department who are eminently qualified in a clinical specialty. The award of the "A" prefix is determined by the Army Surgeon General's Classification Board on an individual basis.

11 Dec 1962 Lt. Col. Isabel S. Paulson became the first Army nurse to be assigned to the Office of the Deputy Chief of Staff for Personnel (DCSPER),

Department of the Army, and detailed to the U.S. Army General Staff to assist in coordinating the recruitment of nurses for the Army.

1963 Lt. Cols. Ruth P. Satterfield, Sadye T. Travers, and Mercedes M. Fischer were the first three Army nurses awarded the "A" prefix to the MOS by the Surgeon General. Colonel Satterfield received the "A" prefix in anesthesia, Colonel Travers in operating room, and Colonel Fischer in Army health nursing.

1963 Blochberger Terrace, a residence for women officers at Fort Leavenworth, Kansas, was named in honor of Lt. Col. Irene C. Blochberger, ANC, of Leavenworth, Kansas. Colonel Blochberger died in 1953 after more than twenty-one years of dedicated service with the United States Army.

1963 Gardiner Hall, a residence for nurses at the United States Army Hospital, Fort Wainwright, Alaska, was named in honor of 2d Lt. Ruth M. Gardiner, ANC. Lieutenant Gardiner, a flight nurse, was killed in a plane crash in Alaska on 25 July 1943 while on an air evacuation mission.

28 Feb 1963 Operation NIGHTINGALE, an intensive nationwide recruitment plan, was initiated by the Department of the Army to stimulate public awareness of the role of the Army nurse and to explain the Army's need for approximately 2,000 nurses.

6 May 1963 Authorization for direct appointment was granted to permit civilian nurses to be commissioned, placed on active duty, and initially assigned to their choice of designated Army hospitals in the continental United States. This authorization was later revised to include designated Army hospitals in overseas commands.

Jul 1963 Army nurses served in the hospital unit which was dispatched to Skopje, Yugoslavia, to aid the victims of a severe earthquake. The 8th Evacuation Hospital sent a 120-bed unit, with thirty nurses, from the Seventh U.S. Army, USAREUR (Germany), to participate in relief operations during July and August.

15 Aug 1963 Lt. Col. Jeanne M. Treacy was the first Army Nurse Corps officer on active duy to attend the Associate Course at the Command and General Staff College, Fort Leavenworth, Kansas.

31 Aug 1963 Col. Margaret Harper, Chief of the Army Nurse Corps, retired. Colonel Harper was the recipient of many honors, including the Legion of Merit upon retirement. Brig. Gen. Conn L. Milburn, Jr., the Deputy Surgeon General, presented the award at a ceremony sponsored by the Lions Club and held in Colonel Harper's hometown of Potomac, Illinois. Others in attendance during the observance of Colonel Margaret Harper Day on 15 September 1963 included the Honorable Leslie Arends, Representative from Illinois; the Deputy Commanding General, Fifth U.S. Army; Army Nurse Corps officers from the Office of the Surgeon General, Second and Fifth U.S. Armies; and members of the Fifth U.S. Army Band.

31 Aug 1963 Army Nurse Corps strength was 2,928: Regular Army, 956; reserve officers on active duty, 1,972. Army Nurse Corps officers were on duty in Army medical treatment facilities in the continental United States, Alaska, Hawaii, Japan, Puerto Rico, Republic of Korea, Thailand, Okinawa, Turkey, Republic of Vietnam, Iran, Ethiopia, Germany, France, and Italy. Approximately fourteen hundred Department of the Army civilian registered nurses were employed to supplement the Army nurses in Army medical treatment facilities worldwide.

1 Sep 1963 Col. Mildred Irene Clark became the twelfth Chief of the Army Nurse Corps.

22 Jan 1964 The minimum age of dependents of women nurses seeking appointment in the Army Nurse Corps Reserve was lowered from eighteen to fifteen years upon approval of request for waiver. The restriction on the minimum age of dependents was not removed until 16 July 1971.

27 Mar 1964 Army nurses participated in relief operations during March and April to aid the victims of a violent earthquake in Alaska. Eleven Army nurses were sent with a medical team from Madigan Army Hospital, Tacoma, Washington, to augment the 64th Field Hospital at Fort Richardson, just outside Anchorage.

1 May 1964 Walter Reed Army Institute of Nursing (WRAIN), Walter Reed Army Medical Center, was established as a class II activity under the jurisdiction of the Surgeon General in cooperation with the University of Maryland School of Nursing, with the academic aspects of the program under the jurisdiction of the university. Maj. Iladene H. Filer was appointed Administrative Director. The program initially provided financial assistance to 135 qualified high school graduates who desired to complete a four-year program in nursing. Upon completion of the program, a bachelor of science degree in nursing was conferred by the University of Maryland. Following state licensure, participants were commissioned as second lieutenants in the U.S. Army Reserve and obligated to serve on active duty for three years. (On 6 January 1975, a Department of the Army message announced that the WRAIN program was being restructured from the existing four-year program to a program limited to the final two years of study leading to a bachelor's degree in nursing. In April 1975, it was announced that recruitment for the program was suspended pending a Department of Defense study of the program. WRAIN was officially closed 30 June 1978.)

Jul 1964 Margaret E. Bailey was promoted to lieutenant colonel after twenty years of service, becoming the first African American nurse to be so honored. In 1969 she was assigned as Health Manpower Training Specialist to the Job Corps Health Office, Department of Labor, and in January 1970 she was promoted to colonel, again the first black nurse to hold that rank.

8 Sep 1964 The U.S. Army exhibit, "The Privilege of Service," honoring officers of the Army Nurse Corps and the Army Medical Specialist Corps (dietitians, physical therapists, and occupational therapists) was unveiled as a permanent display on the Medical Balcony of the Museum of Science and Industry, Chicago, Illinois.

Nov 1964 The Pennsylvania Hospital School of Nursing for Men in Philadelphia had the largest single number of male student nurses to join the Army. Seven male nurses who participated in the Army Student Nurse Program were commissioned as a group into the Army Nurse Corps.

15 Dec 1964 Requirements for the initial appointment of women officers in the Regular Army were revised to permit married applicants to be appointed.

2 Feb 1965 The Army Nurse Corps sponsored an essay contest to commemorate the sixty-fourth anniversary of the Corps. The topic was "What Army Nursing Means to Me in 1965." First award in the active duty category went to Maj. Maude M. Smith, Chief, Nursing Service, 44th Surgical Hospital, Korea; second place in the active duty category went to Capt. Nina West, ANC Counselor from Cincinnati, Ohio; first award in the Army Student Nurse Program category went to Rita Kay Clark of Mount Carmel, Illinois, a junior at Evansville College, Indiana.

Apr 1965 With the rapid buildup of American forces in Vietnam, Army nurses were dispatched with medical units to support the fighting forces. The 8th Field Hospital, Nha Trang, had been the only United States Army hospital in-country for three years. The 3d Field Hospital, Saigon, was the first to arrive during the buildup. Maj. Edith M. Nuttall, of Montesano, Washington, served as the first Chief Nurse of the 3d Field Hospital from 23 April 1965 to 22 April 1966.

24 Apr 1965 Dominican Republic Crisis. Medical units of the United States armed forces were sent to the Dominican Republic to participate in the Inter-American Peace Forces' restoration of peaceful order. Several United States Army medical and paramedical units had been alerted to augment the

15th Field Hospital in support of the 82d Airborne Division. Capt. Leon R. Moore, ANC, arrived at San Isidro with Company D of the 307th Medical Battalion at 0645 on 30 April. Captain Moore began organizing the clearing station, and it was in full operational status by 1600 on 30 April. By 3 May 1965, Army nurses from Fort Bragg, North Carolina, and other posts had joined the staff of the 15th Field Hospital. The last medical detachment left for the United States on 19 September 1966.

9 Aug 1965 The Department of the Army announced a policy whereby registered nurses qualified in surgical nursing and those certified by the American Association of Nurse Anesthetists could volunteer for direct appointment in the Army Nurse Corps and assignment with U.S. Army medical units in Vietnam following the basic orientation course at the Medical Field Service School, Brooke Army Medical Center, Fort Sam Houston, Texas.

15 Sep 1965 Lt. Col. Margaret G. Clarke of Arab, Alabama, became the first Chief Nurse, Office of the Surgeon, U.S. Army, Vietnam (USARV). Before her assignment to USARV headquarters, Colonel Clarke was appointed on 3 February as the Nurse Consultant, Office of the Surgeon, U.S. Army Support Command, Vietnam (USASCV), an additional duty to her primary function as Chief Nurse of the 8th Field Hospital, Nha Trang.

31 Dec 1965 There were 215 Army Nurse Corps officers on duty in field, evacuation, and mobile Army surgical hospitals in Vietnam.

11 Jan 1966 The Warrant Officer Nurse Program was developed at the onset of the military buildup in Southeast Asia to assist in meeting the rapidly expanded personnel requirements for military nursing services in the Army. Graduates of two-year associate degree programs in nursing education were authorized appointment as warrant officers in the Army of the United States with concurrent call to active duty for a period of two years (DA Message 746525). WO1 Edward J. Dabkowski of New Britain, Connecticut, was the first ANC member appointed as a warrant officer. More than ninety registered nurses served as warrant officers (ANC) before the program was suspended with the expiration of DA Circular 601–20 on 3 April 1968.

Feb 1966 Nearly 300 military nurses, both men and women, of the Army, Navy, and Air Force were serving in Vietnam. The Army had over 200, the Navy 39, including 29 serving aboard the hospital ship *Repose*, and the Air Force 37, not including flight nurses assigned aboard medical air evacuation aircraft moving the sick and wounded to hospitals in the United States.

Apr 1966 Special Call Number 38 for the draft of 900 male nurses was issued. In this call, the Department of Defense requested 700 nurses for the Army and 200 for the Navy. The health services requirements of the increased active military strength and the treatment needs of casualties from Southeast Asia necessitated this action. This call yielded 27 warrant officers and 124 commissioned officers for the Army Nurse Corps.

May 1966 Col. Margaret G. Clarke was selected as U.S. Army Nurse of the Year for 1965.

Jul 1966 The first brother and sister to serve together in the Army Nurse Corps were 2d Lt. Terrance Friedhoff and Maj. Erla Friedhoff. The Friedhoffs were assigned to the 249th Army General Hospital, Camp Drake, Japan.

30 Sep 1966 Public Law 89–609, 89th Congress, authorized commissions in the Regular Army for male nurses. Mrs. Frances P. Bolton, Representative from Ohio, had first introduced such legislation, H.R. 8135, in 1961 and an identical bill, H.R. 1034, in January 1963. Mrs. Bolton again introduced the legislation, H.R. 420, on 4 January 1965; Samuel S. Stratton, Representative from New York, introduced identical legislation, H.R. 8158, on 13 May 1965.

1967 An ANC officer was assigned as Nurse Consultant, Consultant Division, Professional Service Directorate, Office of the Surgeon General. In addition to consultant duties, this officer provided liaison between ANC consultants and the Office of the Surgeon General and other Army agencies requiring ANC consultant services.

2 Feb 1967 Capt. Linda Anne Bowman received the first annual Dr. Anita Newcomb McGee Award presented by the National Society of the Daughters of the American Revolution. Dr. McGee became known as the founder of the Army Nurse Corps after the legislation she wrote eventually became a part of the Army Reorganization Act which was passed by the Congress and established the Army Nurse Corps on 2 February 1901. (See Appendix C.)

5 May 1967 Lt. Col. Patricia T. Murphy, ANC, was the first Army Nurse Corps officer to receive the Pace Award, presented annually in the name of Frank Pace, former Secretary of the Army, for a contribution of outstanding significance to the Army during the calendar year. The award was presented to Colonel Murphy for her outstanding contributions to patient care and treatment aspects of the Medical Unit, Self-contained, Transportable (MUST) Project while assigned to the MUST Project Office, United States Army Medical Research and Development Command, Office of the Surgeon General. The award was presented in the Office of the Secretary of the Army by the former Secretary of the Army, the Honorable Frank Pace. In 1966, the 45th Surgical Hospital, the first MUST hospital in Vietnam, became operational. This inflatable rubber shelter with integral electrical power, air conditioning, heating, hot and cold water, and waste disposal could be transported by truck, helicopter, or cargo aircraft.

16 Aug 1967 Maj. Doris S. Frazier was the first Army Nurse Corps officer selected to attend the resident course at the Command and General Staff College, Fort Leavenworth, Kansas.

31 Aug 1967 Col. Mildred Irene Clark completed the statutory four-year appointment as Chief of the Army Nurse Corps. She served as Special Assistant to the Director, Personnel and Training for Nursing Activities, Office of the Surgeon General, from 1 September 1967 until her retirement on 11 October 1967. Colonel Clark was the recipient of many honors, including the Distinguished Service Medal awarded for eminently meritorious service while serving as Chief of the Army Nurse Corps, and the University of Minnesota's Outstanding Achievement Award. She was honored by her hometown of Clarkton, North Carolina, on Irene Clark Day.

1 Sep 1967 Col. Anna Mae Hays became the thirteenth Chief of the Army Nurse Corps.

8 Nov 1967 Public Law 90–130, passed by the 90th Congress and signed by President Lyndon B. Johnson, was entitled "A Bill to Amend Titles 10, 32, and 37, United States Code, to Remove Restrictions on the Careers of Female Officers in the Army, Navy, Air Force and Marine Corps, and for Other Purposes." This legislation authorized promotion consideration of Army Nurse Corps, Army Medical Specialist Corps, and Women's Army Corps officers under the same promotion procedures applicable to men in the Regular Army.

Jul 1968 Kay Lemieux graduated from nursing school, becoming the third daughter of Mr. and Mrs. Robert Lemieux of Terre Haute, Indiana, to enter the Army Nurse Corps through the Army Student Nurse Program. The first daughter, 1st Lt. Elizabeth Lemieux, served in Vietnam and was an ANC Counselor. The second daughter, Capt. Mary Ann Lemieux, was serving with the 7th Surgical Hospital in Vietnam.

Fall 1968 The Medical Command in Japan also cared for the sick and wounded from Southeast Asia. There was only one hospital in Japan in 1965 which had 100 available beds. By 1966 there were four hospitals, including the 7th Field Hospital (400 beds), the 249th General Hospital (1,000 beds), and the 106th General Hospital (1,000 beds). The U.S. Army Hospital at Camp Zama was increased from its original 100 to 700 beds. There were 280 nurses assigned to the command during 1968.

9 Oct 1968 Lt. Col. M. Sue Walker, USARAN, arrived in Vietnam to serve as the Chief Nurse of the 312th Evacuation Hospital, Chu Lai, the first and only U.S. Army Reserve evacuation hospital in Vietnam. From their home station in Winston-Salem, North Carolina, hospital personnel were ordered to active duty on 11 April 1968, later mobilized at Fort Benning, Georgia, and deployed to Vietnam on 25 September. Army nurses were assigned to seven of the eleven USAR medical units ordered to active duty on 11 April 1968. They were deployed to Vietnam with the following medical units beginning on 19 September: 305th Surgical Detachment (Pennsylvania); 378th Neurosurgical Detachment (Indiana); 312th Evacuation Hospital (North Carolina); 313th and 889th Surgical Detachments (Virginia). Beginning on 13 October 1968, the 74th Field Hospital (New York) and the 311th Field Hospital (Ohio) deployed. All of the USAR medical units returned to reserve status in January 1970.

19 Nov 1968 Seven additional Army Nurse Corps officers were appointed consultants to the Surgeon General in clinical nursing specialties and in nursing education and research. Before that time, ANC officers were assigned as consultants in Army health nursing, operating room, and anesthesia.

1969 Majs. Maria Segura and Nilda Carreras were assigned to assist with nursing educational programs for six months at Guardia National Hospital, Nicaragua.

30 Jun 1969 The Department of Nursing became the organizational title for the nursing activities within U.S. Army hospitals.

Sep 1969 A cooperative graduate program was established by the U.S. Army's Tripler General Hospital and the University of Hawaii. Graduates of this program received a master's degree in nursing with a major in biophysical pathology and certification to practice anesthesiology nursing. Six ANC officers graduated from this program.

11 Nov 1969 On Veterans Day, the Lane Recovery Suite at Fitzsimons General Hospital, Denver, Colorado, was formally dedicated in memory of 1st Lt. Sharon A. Lane, ANC, of Canton, Ohio. Lieutenant Lane's first assignment as an Army Nurse Corps officer had been at Fitzsimons General Hospital. She died on 8 June 1969 of shrapnel wounds received during an enemy rocket attack while on duty at the 312th Evacuation Hospital in Chu Lai, Republic of Vietnam. Lieutenant Lane was the only Army nurse killed as a result of enemy action during the Vietnam War. The Bronze Star Medal and the Purple Heart were awarded posthumously. The Dr. Anita Newcomb McGee Award was presented posthumously by the National Society of the Daughters of the American Revolution on 22 April 1970.

Jan 1970 Army regulations were changed to permit waivers and allow retention of married female officers who became pregnant while on active duty. Maternity leave in the form of ordinary leave and excess leave was authorized.

Feb 1970 First Lt. John D. Ford became the Army's first anesthesia student to be commissioned under the Registered Nurse Student Program (RNSP). Lieutenant Ford was one of 1,000 male nurses serving in the Army Nurse Corps.

11 Jun 1970 Col. Anna Mae Hays, Chief, Army Nurse Corps, was promoted to brigadier general. She was the first nurse in the history of the American military to attain general officer rank.

Sep 1970 Insurrection in Amman, Jordan. The International Red Cross requested the assistance of an all-male contingent of Army Nurse Corps officers. Sixteen men were airlifted to Jordan with the 32d Surgical Hospital, USARMEDCOMEUR (Germany), to participate in relief operations during September and October.

Sep 1970 Lt. Col. Madeline Bader, Chief of Clinical Nursing of Psychiatry and Neurology, played an active role in planning and implementing Project Crisis Awareness and Management (CAM) at Walter Reed Army Medical Center. The program was designed to assist terminally ill patients and their families, as well as staff members, to cope with serious medical problems and terminal illness. Colonel Bader used psychiatric nurses in the emergency room and oncology service to assist anxious relatives and friends and to serve as a role model to the staff. Colonel Bader was awarded the coveted "A" prefix for continued excellence and competence in one's field.

1971 Lt. Col. Lyndoll L. Wells was assigned as Nursing Consultant in the Facilities Branch of the Directorate of Plans, Supply and Operations, Office of the Surgeon General, in Washington, D.C. This was the first time a nurse was assigned to the branch to assist with planning of medical facilities.

22 Feb 1971 A task force of Army Nurse Corps consultants was convened to initiate planning for the AN–CP (Army Nursing–Contemporary Practice) Program. A coordinated plan was developed for advanced training in clinical specialties to prepare nurse clinicians for specific primary nursing roles.

16 Jul 1971 Restriction on the age of dependents (not under fifteen years of age) of women nurses seeking appointment in the Army Nurse Corps Reserve was removed by authority of a Department of the Army message issued in May 1971 and Army Regulations No. 601–139 published in July 1971.

31 Aug 1971 Brig. Gen. Anna Mae Hays completed the statutory four-year appointment as Chief of the Army Nurse Corps. General Hays was the recipient of many honors, including the Distinguished Service Medal presented by General William C. Westmoreland, Chief of Staff, U.S. Army.

1 Sep 1971 Brig. Gen. Lillian Dunlap, the second Army Nurse Corps officer to serve in the grade of general officer, was promoted and sworn in as the fourteenth Chief of the Army Nurse Corps.

Jan 1972 The first students entered the Army Nurse Corps Clinician Program to prepare as nurse clinicians in ambulatory care, obstetrics-gynecology, and pediatric nursing. The first nurse clinicians were graduated in June 1972 and assigned to selected Army hospitals where the outpatient workload had increased significantly. These clinicians progressively assumed increased responsibility for the assessment, treatment, teaching, and follow-up care of patients with common minor and chronic health problems.

1 Feb 1972 Helen G. McClelland, one of only three Army nurses ever to receive the Distinguished Service Cross (an award second in rank only to the Medal of Honor, the highest award in combat), took part in the unveiling of a display of her World War I uniform, medals, and helmet at the Medical Museum, Armed Forces Institute of Pathology. The display included Miss McClelland's handkerchief and nurse's cap riddled with holes ripped out by German bomb fragments. Miss McClelland was on duty at British Casualty Clearing Station No. 61, on the front line in Belgium, when the hospital was bombed by the Germans on 17 August 1917. In an extraordinary act of heroism, without concern for her personal safety, Miss McClelland aided the wounded and was credited with saving the life of another American nurse, Miss Beatrice McDonald, while the hospital area was still under fire. Miss McClelland was also recognized by Great Britain with the award of the British Royal Red Cross, First Class. Field Marshal Douglas Haig included her in his list of those who served with great gallantry on the Western Front.

May 1972 Capt. Shirley Cotton, ANC Counselor for Los Angeles, was the first Army nurse assigned to accompany a United Service Organization (USO) troupe to Vietnam. She spent a week on tour with Sammy Davis Jr's group.

1 Jul 1972 Col. Margaret E. Bailey, USA (Ret.), was designated as Consultant to the Surgeon General to promote increased participation by minority group members in Army Nurse Corps recruitment programs.

Sep 1972 A Nurse-Midwifery Service, the first such separate service, was started at Ireland Army Hospital, Fort Knox, Kentucky. Capt. Barbara Schroeder was the first nurse-midwife assigned to this service. Lt. Col. Mary G. Mulqueen, ANC Consultant to the Surgeon General in Maternity Nursing, was assigned to the service in February 1973.

Oct 1972 A bachelor's degree with a major in nursing or evidence of progress toward such a degree became a requirement for appointment to the Regular Army.

1 Mar 1973 Lt. Col. Geraldene Felton, Lt. Col. Phyllis Verhonick (Ret.), and Lt. Col. Harriet Werley (Ret.) were elected as Fellows of the American Academy of Nursing. The academy was established to enhance the quality of health care in the United States by exploring broad problems confronting nursing and the health field.

29 Mar 1973 The last of more than five thousand nurses departed from the Republic of Vietnam two months after the cease-fire. Lt. Col. Marion L. Minter of Carlisle, Pennsylvania, was the last Chief Nurse of Vietnam. She served in the dual role as Nurse Consultant to the Headquarters, U.S. Army Health Services Group, Vietnam, and as Chief Nurse of the U.S. Army Hospital, Saigon (formerly 3d Field Hospital), from 28 August 1972 to 29 March 1973.

During the eleven-year period between March 1962 and March 1973, peak strength in South Vietnam reached over nine hundred Army Nurse Corps officers in 1969. Nine Army nurses died while serving in Vietnam. The only nurse to die as a result of hostile fire was 1st Lt. Sharon A. Lane, of Canton, Ohio. Lieutenant Lane died of shrapnel wounds during an enemy rocket attack on 8 June 1969 while on duty at the 312th Evacuation Hospital, Chu Lai. Second Lts. Carol Ann Drazba and Elizabeth Jones died in a helicopter crash on 18 February 1966 near Saigon. Capt. Eleanor G. Alexander, and 1st Lts. Jerome E. Olmstead, Hedwig D. Orlowski, and Kenneth R. Shoemaker died in a plane crash near Qui Nhon on 30 November 1967. The four nurses had been on temporary duty assignments with the 71st Evacuation Hospital, Pleiku, and were en route to the 67th and 85th Evacuation Hospitals when the plane crashed. Second Lt. Pamela D. Donovan of the 85th Evacuation Hospital died in country of disease on 8 July 1968. Lt. Col. Annie Ruth Graham, a veteran of World War II and service in Japan during the Korean War and Chief Nurse of the 91st Evacuation Hospital, died of illness 14 August 1968 after evacuation to Japan.

1 Apr 1973 The United States Army Health Services Command (HSC) became operational at Fort Sam Houston, Texas, as part of the general reorganization of the Army. The command provided a single manager for the entire Army health care and educational system within the continental United States. In

1974, the command assumed responsibilities for Army health care in Alaska, Hawaii, and the Canal Zone. Maj. Gen. Spurgeon Neel, MC, was selected as the first Commander of the United States Army Health Services Command.

Twelve Army Nurse Corps officers were assigned to the command headquarters, with Col. Virginia L. Brown as the first Chief of the Nursing Division. Lt. Col. Patricia A. Silvestre and Maj. Claire M. McQuail were the first Army nurses to be assigned to the Office of the Inspector General (IG) as members of the IG Team, HSC. The inspection activities by the Army Nurse Corps officers were directed primarily toward evaluation of mission performance of hospital departments of nursing and the quality of care provided to patients.

11 Jun 1973 Lt. Col. Doris S. Frazier was the first Army Nurse Corps officer to graduate from the Army War College.

Aug 1973 Lt. Col. Connie L. Slewitzke, ANC, served as class president during the resident course at the Command and General Staff College, the first time a woman had held this office.

23 Oct 1973 Brig. Gen. Lillian Dunlap became the first woman in the history of the United States Army to serve as president of a Department of the Army officer promotion board.

Jan 1974 Capts. Roberta Randall and Marilyn Rees were the first two students to enter the U.S. Army University of Kentucky Nurse-Midwifery Program. This was a collaborative, contractual arrangement between the Army and the University of Kentucky.

In May 1975, the degree of Master of Science in Nursing was conferred by the University of Kentucky College of Nursing and Captains Randall and Rees were among the first graduates. Brig. Gen. Lillian Dunlap, Chief, Army Nurse Corps, gave the commencement address before the graduating class of the University of Kentucky College of Nursing. By February 1980, eighteen Army nurses had completed the program.

2 Mar 1974 Lt. Col. Lawrence W. Scheffner was promoted to the grade of colonel in the Army of the United States. Colonel Scheffner thus became the first man in the Army Nurse Corps to serve in the grade of colonel.

Oct 1974 For the first time, Army Nurse Corps officers could receive graduate-level credit for any one of five nurse clinician courses. Selected Army nurses who met the graduate school entrance requirements for the University of Texas System School of Nursing and successfully completed the clinician course received sixteen semester hours of academic credit that could be applied to a master's program. The five courses and the Army hospitals designated to provide the clinical courses were:

Nurse Clinician Ambulatory Care Course
Hays Army Hospital, Fort Ord, California
Martin Army Hospital, Fort Benning, Georgia

Nurse Clinician Intensive Care Course
Brooke Army Medical Center, Fort Sam Houston, Texas
Fitzsimons Army Medical Center, Denver, Colorado

Nurse Clinician Pediatric Course
Fitzsimons Army Medical Center, Denver, Colorado
Madigan Army Medical Center, Tacoma, Washington

Nurse Clinician Obstetrics-Gynecology Nursing Course
Womack Army Hospital, Fort Bragg, North Carolina

Nurse Clinician Psychiatric–Mental Health Course
Walter Reed Army Medical Center, Washington, D.C.

2 Feb 1975 The former Chiefs of the Army Nurse Corps were honored on the seventy-fourth anniversary of the Corps. A memorial service was held at the Walter Reed Army Medical Center Chapel. A brunch and reception followed at the WRAMC Officers Club. The honored guests present and their tenure of office were:

Col. Ruby F. Bryant	1 Oct 51–30 Sep 55
Col. Inez Haynes	1 Oct 55–31 Aug 59
Col. Margaret Harper	1 Sep 59–31 Aug 63
Col. Mildred I. Clark	1 Sep 63–31 Aug 67
Brig. Gen. Anna Mae Hays	1 Sep 67–31 Aug 71

Also honored but unable to attend because of illness was Col. Mary G. Phillips, Chief of the Army Nurse Corps from 1 October 1947 to 30 September 1951. The guest speaker was Lt. Gen. Richard R. Taylor, the Surgeon General.

3 Feb 1975 Four former Chiefs of the Army Nurse Corps, Cols. Ruby F. Bryant, Inez Haynes, Margaret Harper, and Mildred I. Clark, and the then incumbent Chief of the Army Nurse Corps, Brig. Gen. Lillian Dunlap, took part in a workshop at the Historical Unit, USAMEDD, Fort Detrick, Maryland. Col. John Lada, MSC, Director, hosted the meeting. Procedures were developed for gathering and centralizing a comprehensive data bank of ANC information and memorabilia in the continuing effort to fully document the history of the Army Nurse Corps.

Mar 1975 From 1963 to this date, thirty-eight Army Nurse Corps officers had been awarded the "A" prefix to the MOS designation in one of seven clinical specialties:

3431	Community Health Nursing
3437	Psychiatric/Mental Health Nursing
3442	Pediatric Nursing
3443	Operating Room Nursing
3445	Anesthesiology Nursing
3446	Obstetrics and Gynecology Nursing
3448	Medical-Surgical Nursing

25 Apr 1975 Operation NEW LIFE. Federal and civilian agencies helped in the evacuation and care of more than 130,000 Indochinese refugees before and following the end of the Vietnam War on 7 May 1975. Army Medical Department personnel joined the 45th Support Group deployed from Hawaii to Orote Point, Guam. Lt. Col. Jeanne Hoppe was the Chief Nurse on Guam. Four refugee centers were chosen in the continental United States: Camp Pendleton, California; Eglin Air Force Base, Florida; Fort Chaffee, Arkansas; and Indiantown Gap Military Reservation, Pennsylvania.

On 29 April, Army nurses were dispatched to join other Army Medical Department personnel at Fort Chaffee, Arkansas. Lt. Col. Velma J. Barkley was the chief nurse. On 1 May, the title of this humanitarian relief operation was changed to Operation NEW ARRIVALS. On 25 May, the hospital at Indiantown Gap became operational to provide medical support for more than fifteen thousand refugees. Lt. Col. Vera A. Nolfe was the chief nurse.

May 1975 Col. Madelyn N. Parks, Chief, Department of Nursing, Walter Reed Army Medical Center, was nominated for promotion to brigadier general and selected to succeed Brig. Gen. Lillian Dunlap as Chief, Army Nurse Corps, on 1 September 1975.

Jun 1975 Capt. Jeanne Picariello was the first woman and to date the only nurse to participate as a member of the U.S. Army Pentathalon Team. She participated on the team between 1975 and 1978.

14 Jun 1975 On the two hundredth anniversary of the United States Army, Brig. Gen. Lillian Dunlap, Chief of the Army Nurse Corps, took part in the United States Army Bicentennial Memorial Service at Arlington National Cemetery. General Dunlap led the congregation in the responsive reading. The memorial address was given by General Fred C. Weyand, Chief of Staff, United States Army. The hymn, "Mighty Is Our Army," written by Sfc. Ralph L. Bowerman especially for the Army's Bicentennial observance, was introduced for the first time by the United States Army Band and Chorus.

18 Jun 1975 The Republic of Korea Presidential Unit Citation was awarded to the 43d Surgical Hospital (Mobile Army) for meritorious service rendered to the Republic of Korea for nearly twenty-five years—from July 1950 to 28 February 1975. As the first and last U.S. Army surgical hospital in Korea, the 43d Surgical Hospital was cited for outstanding medical care and service for the members of the United States Army and the United Nations forces and Korean patients.

1 Jan 1976 Length of long tours in overseas areas was changed from twenty-four months to thirty-six months for single females. This equalized the length of tours for single males and females.

Mar 1976 The authorized ANC strength in Army Reserve troop program units was increased from approximately 1,900 to over 5,100 officers. In February 1980 the United States Army Recruiting Command took over the responsibility for recruitment of the nurses for the reserve units.

Apr 1976 The Division of Nursing at the Walter Reed Army Institute of Research transferred to the Department of Nursing, Walter Reed Army Medical Center. It was designated the Nursing Research Service and continued its focus in the area of clinical nursing research.

12 May 1976 The United States Army Health Clinic at Fort Hamilton, New York, was dedicated to 2d Lt. Ellen G. Ainsworth. She was killed on the Anzio beachhead on 10 February 1944 and received the Silver Star posthumously.

Jun 1976 Lt. Col. Clara Adams-Ender was the first nurse and first African American female to receive the Master of Military Art and Science degree from the Command and General Staff College, Fort Leavenworth, Kansas.

Oct 1976 A bachelor's degree with a major in nursing became a requirement for accession to active duty.

Nov 1976 The first organizational meeting of the Retired Army Nurse Corps Association was held. RANCA was incorporated the following year and held its first biennial convention in San Antonio, Texas, 14–15 April 1978, with 326 registrants present.

Spring 1977 USAR Unit Chief Nurses conferences were held at Fort Meade, Maryland; Fort Sam Houston, Texas; and San Francisco, California. This was the first time the USAR Chief Nurses had an opportunity to discuss common problems and to share information directly with members of the Surgeon General's Office; the Nurse Staff Adviser, Office of the Chief, Army Reserve; and the Chief Nurse, Office of the Surgeon, Forces Command.

Conferences were held again in 1979, and it was planned that they be held every two years.

Aug 1977 Two new titles were adopted to replace the previously used title of Nurse Clinician. These new titles, Nurse Practitioner and Clinical Nurse Specialist, reflected the greater utilization of Army Nurse Corps officers in expanded roles. The nurse practitioner must be a graduate of a six-month course in a given specialty and work primarily in the clinic environment, whereas the clinical nurse specialist must have a master's degree in nursing and perform in the expanded role within specific clinical areas of an inpatient facility.

Sep 1977 All new baccalaureate of science in nursing graduate accessions were commissioned as second lieutenants.

Oct 1977 Lt. Col. Margie O. Burt, Certified Registered Nurse Anesthetist, was selected to initiate the Reserve Component Personnel and Administration Center (RCPAC), St. Louis, Missouri, Officer Personnel Management System (OPMS) program for ANC officers. A second ANC officer, Capt. Patsy Bramley, was assigned one and a half years later to assist Colonel Burt.

The OPMS program included all ANC control group and troop unit reserve officers. Opportunities open to the ANC officer included professional development by enrollment in correspondence courses, attendance at schools for short and long courses, assignment to units, participation in counterpart training with an active Army installation, and personnel counseling.

Nov 1977 Brig. Gen. Madelyn N. Parks, Chief, Army Nurse Corps, visited the People's Republic of China for four weeks. The American Nurses' Association invited twenty nursing leaders to visit Chinese health care facilities, work areas, and homes to better understand the Chinese people and health care systems. The group visited Peking, Chengchow, Kaifeng, Wusih, Shanghai, and Canton.

14 Nov 1977 The Northeast Regional Accrediting Committee of the American Nurses' Association accredited the Army Nurse Corps as a provider and approver of continuing education for nursing programs. These programs are offered at individual posts, regional Army medical centers, and at the U.S. Army Academy of Health Sciences.

Jun 1978 Maj. Janet Rexrode served as the Army's Senior White House Social Aide. White House Social Aides are a corps of 25–35 officers who welcome guests to the White House in the name of the First Family. Being an aide is a collateral, voluntary duty. Major Rexrode was a doctoral student in nursing service at The Catholic University of America at the time she held this position.

3 Jun 1978 The final Walter Reed Army Institute of Nursing (WRAIN) commissioning ceremony was held with ninety-one graduate nurses commissioned as first lieutenants. At this ceremony the WRAIN unit flag and crest were retired and donated to Army nurses for future display in the Army Medical Museum. During its eleven years, five ANC officers served as WRAIN's Director: Lt. Col. Iladene H. Filer (1964–1967), Lt. Col. Margaret Ewen (1967–1968), Col. Drusilla Poole (1968–1974), Lt. Col. Billie J. Barcus (1974–1976), and Col. Hazel W. Johnson (1976–1978).

18 Aug 1978 The Army Nurse Corps Nursing Research Advisory Board (ANC-NRAB) was established to advise and assist the Chief of the Army Nurse Corps in establishing nursing research priorities and to monitor the progress of nursing research throughout the Army Medical Department. The Nursing Research Service, Department of Nursing, Walter Reed Army Medical Center, was responsible for monitoring and coordinating research ideas and for providing research proposal assistance to Army nurses worldwide. Other ANC assignments involving nursing research were with the Health Care Division, Academy of Health Sciences, Health Services Command, Fort Sam Houston, Texas, and the Preventive Medicine Division, Walter Reed Army Institute of Research.

1979 Majs. Cecil B. Drain and Susan B. Shipley coauthored the first text on recovery room procedures and techniques written wholly by nurses. The book, entitled *The Recovery Room*, was published by W. B. Saunders Co., Philadelphia, in 1979.

Jan 1979 Lt. Col. Betty Brice, Obstetrical/Gynecologic Consultant, accompanied the 1st Division to Europe during Exercise REFORGER '79 to assess the medical needs of women at different levels of the division.

Jun 1979 Col. Hazel W. Johnson was nominated for promotion to brigadier general and selected to succeed Brig. Gen. Madelyn N. Parks as Chief, Army Nurse Corps, on 1 September 1979. Colonel Johnson received many honors, including the Legion of Merit. She received her doctorate in educational administration in 1978 from Catholic University. She was the first African American female general officer in the Department of Defense.

Oct 1979 Maj. Janet Southby, Chief, Nursing Research Service, WRAMC, received the 1979 Federal Nursing Service Award. The award, presented annually by the Association of Military Surgeons of the United States, honors the best essay on a subject that advances professional nursing.

Nov 1979 The initial draft of Standards of Nursing Practice was issued for implementation and evaluation at all Army hospitals.

Jan 1980 Maj Sharon Richie became the first Army nurse to provide clinical liaison with the Alcohol and Drug Abuse Program Consultants Office to coordinate the medical aspects of the Army's alcohol and drug abuse prevention and control programs. In July 1980 she was reassigned to the office of Brig. Gen. William Louisell, Deputy Assistant Secretary of Defense for Drug and Alcohol Abuse Prevention as the Assistant Director for Education and Rehabilitation.

Mar 1980 By this date more than 3,660—approximately 95 percent—of the Army nurses on active duty had a baccalaureate degree or higher in nursing or a related career field; of that number 608 had earned master's degrees and 8 had their doctorate. There were 3,856 Army Nurse Corps officers on active duty in the United States, Hawaii, Alaska, Panama, Japan, Okinawa, the Republic of Korea, Germany, Italy, and Belgium.

31 May 1980 The authorized strength for the Army Nurse Corps in United States Army Reserve medical units was 5,682. There were 3,183 United States Army Reserve (USAR) Nurse Corps officers assigned to paid drill spaces and participating in training programs. National Guard authorized nurse strength was 661. The assigned strength was 626.

Spring 1980 Fifty-four Army nurses and other Army Medical Department personnel assisted in the evacuation and care of Cuban refugees during Freedom Flotilla, the mass movement of some 125,000 Cuban refugees into the United States. The principal refugee camps were established at Fort Chaffee, Arkansas; Fort Indiantown Gap, Pennsylvania; and Fort McCoy, Wisconsin.

Jul 1980 Col. Rosemary McCarthy, ANC Historian, cofounded and became Recording Secretary of the International History of Nursing Society, later known as the American Association for the History of Nursing.

Jul 1980 A Pentagon conference room used by the Secretary of the Army was dedicated to 2d Lt. Ellen G. Ainsworth. She was killed on the Anzio beachhead on 10 February 1944. (See entry for 12 May 1976.)

10 Jul 1980 The Presidential Suite within the Dwight D. Eisenhower Executive Nursing Suite at Walter Reed Army Medical Center was dedicated in memory of Lt. Col. Phyllis J. Verhonick for her outstanding contributions to military nursing research. This suite is used by heads of state and national and foreign military and civilian leaders whose status or position might require extraordinary privacy or security arrangements.

1981 After several years of testing and revision, the Army Nurse Corps Standards of Nursing Practice were published as an official DA Pamphlet (DA PAM 40–5).

Jun 1981 A hospital-based nursing alternative to the traditional Reserve Officers Training Corps (ROTC) summer camp, the Nurse Summer Training Program, was successfully tested in each of the four ROTC Regions at Fort Bragg, North Carolina, Fort Knox, Kentucky, Fort Riley, Kansas, and Fort Lewis, Washington. Twenty-four cadets successfully completed the program.

Jun 1981 The first Phyllis J. Verhonick Nursing Research Symposium was held in San Antonio, Texas. This biennial, one-week course was devoted to research design and methodology and provided a forum for reporting ANC nursing research. Over fifty papers were submitted in competition for the Phyllis J. Verhonick Nursing Research Award. Maj. Susie M. Sherrod was the first recipient for her study related to a patient classification system. (See Appendix F.)

Sep 1981 The Defense Officer Personnel Management Act (DOPMA) affected the grade at which experienced nurses could be accessed. Previously qualified for the rank of captain or major, they now were eligible to enter active duty only as first lieutenants.

Sep 1981 Lt. Col. Ira P. Gunn (Ret.) was named a Fellow of the American Academy of Nursing. She was the first nurse anesthetist to be so honored.

1982 The Chief Nurse Orientation Course was renamed Principles of Advanced Nursing Administration for ANC Officers. The new target population included supervisory-level personnel.

1982 Two ANC officers, Capts. Sandra Yaney and Leslie Dempsey, were assigned to the OTSG Task Force on Fitness. These officers designed and implemented the ODCSPER Corporate Fitness Research Program to help determine Army policy and future initiatives related to health fitness. Capt. Jeanne Picariello was assigned to the Army Physical Fitness Research Institute at the U.S. Army War College, Carlisle, Pennsylvania. The institute was engaged in research and testing senior officer physical fitness and field testing fitness programs Army-wide.

1982 The ANC's Anesthesiology for Nursing Course became affiliated with the State University of New York at Buffalo. Graduates received a Master of Science in Nursing degree with a major in anesthesia. In 1984 this affiliation transferred to Texas Wesleyan College which awarded the Master in Health Sciences degree.

Jan 1982 Maj. Paul Farineau spent three months in Egypt as part of a Project Hope effort to increase the ability of Egyptian physicians and medical technicians to teach emergency care.

Feb 1982 Lt. Col. Charles Bombard was assigned to a military assistance project under the U.S. Army Material Development and Readiness Command (DARCOM) to provide consultation to the Saudi Arabian National Guard and to supervise contractor operations for nursing services in administration of a new 500-bed facility.

Mar 1982 Following the Camp David agreements, three ANC officers, Capt. Patrick M. Schretenthaler, 2d Lt. Paul Escott, and Capt. Delois Daniels accompanied the first contingent of U.S. troops to the Sinai to assist in the operation of two health clinics. They were the first nurses to be assigned to the United Nations Sinai peacekeeping force and provided care to the multinational force and observers, to civilian contract employees, to other civilians in emergencies, and later to nomadic Bedouins.

Jun 1982 First Lt. Jane A. Delano, third Superintendent of the Army Nurse Corps and Director of Nursing Services of the American Red Cross, and Col. Julia C. Stimson, fifth Superintendent of the Army Nurse Corps and past president of the American Nurses' Association, were inducted into the American Nurses' Association Hall of Fame.

Sep 1982 The new hospital at Fort Campbell, Kentucky, was dedicated and named the Colonel Florence A. Blanchfield Army Community Hospital. This was the first permanent U.S. Army hospital named for a female and for a nurse.

Sep 1982 Maj. Sharon Richie was the first Army Medical Department officer to be selected a White House Fellow. She served with the Office of Intergovernmental Affairs, The White House. The program provides an opportunity for selected individuals to work closely in a combined educational and apprentice situation with elected and appointed government officials.

Dec 1982 For the first time in three years a patient was admitted to the U.S. Army Medical Research Institute of Infectious Disease's Special Ward Isolation Suite. This admission provided ANC officers valuable experience in delivering care to a highly infected patient while wearing vinyl positive pressure suits. The Isolation Suite was established to provide care for patients with potentially fatal, high-risk, infectious disease for which routine hospital isolation procedures were inadequate. Army nurses developed and revised isolation procedures as a result of this unique experience.

Dec 1982 Col. Connie L. Slewitzke represented the ANC on a DOD-sponsored trip to the People's Republic of China. The group toured Chinese military medical facilities and educational and research activities.

1983 Majs. Patricia Curry and Elise Gates were assigned as the first ROTC Region Chief Nurses for the First and Fourth ROTC Regions, respectively.

Jan 1983 The first Army Nurse Corps officer to attend the Combat Casualty Care Course (C4) was Maj. Barbara Smith. This ten-day, tri-service effort, designed originally for physicians and conducted at the Academy of Health Sciences and nearby Camp Bullis, Fort Sam Houston, Texas, provided an intensive program of field medical and survival skills.

Feb 1983 Lt. Col. Dorothy Clark was assigned to the 7th Medical Command (MEDCOM), United Kingdom Plans Division, in Burtonwood, England. Her work related to the requirements, locations, and equipment necessary for contingency hospitals.

Mar 1983 Maj. Annette R. Aitcheson, USA Institute of Surgical Research, was deployed to Amman, Jordan, to organize from the nursing point of view the Jordanian Army Burn Treatment Centre by providing job descriptions of nursing staff, training in the development and organization of the nursing staff, and recommendations on policies and procedures in the implementation of Jordan's Burn Treatment Centre.

Apr 1983 The first "Specialty Nursing Standards of Practice for Community Health Nursing" was published as an adjunct to DA Pamphlet 40–5. On 15 May 1986, "Specialty Nursing Standards: Occupational Health Nursing" was added. Occupational health nurses played a major role in the development of a medical module for the Occupational Health Management Information System (OHMIS), which provided guidelines for nurses and physicians in preemployment, administrative, and job-related surveillance examinations.

Jun 1983 Capt. Juan Sandoval was assigned for six months to El Salvador as a member of a humanitarian medical treatment team. He evaluated hospital nursing auxiliary services and health needs within garrison areas and served as a consultant to provide professional assistance and advice to medic instructors.

Jun 1983 Lt. Col. Collette Keyser was the first ANC officer assigned to Health Care Operations of the Surgeon General's Office to participate in the development of Deployable Medical Systems. These modular medical components were part of a quad-service effort to standardize field medical facilities throughout DOD.

Jul 1983 Col. Clara L. Adams-Ender, Chief Nurse of the U.S. Army Recruiting Command (USAREC), was the recipient of the Roy Wilkins Meritorious Service Award presented by the National Association for the Advancement of Colored People (NAACP) at its annual convention in New Orleans, Louisiana.

Jul 1983 Col. Amelia J Carson reported for duty in the Office of the Surgeon, Army National Guard Bureau, as the first Chief Nurse for the Army National Guard.

Jul 1983 The first Field Nursing Course was conducted at the Academy of Health Sciences and Camp Bullis, Texas, to prepare those assigned to field units as training nurses or chief nurses.

Jul 1983 Advance elements of the 41st Combat Support Hospital deployed to Honduras to establish an aid station. The remainder of the hospital arrived in August as part of Exercise AHAUS TARA II to support Joint Task Force–Bravo during field exercises. In addition to providing medical support to soldiers, the hospital staff provided humanitarian assistance and medical training to the Hondurans.

31 Aug 1983 Brig. Gen. Hazel W. Johnson-Brown, sixteenth Chief of the Army Nurse Corps, retired. She had directed the WRAIN program and was Chief Nurse of the 18th Medical Command, Korea, during her career. Upon her retirement she assumed the position of Director of the Division of Government Affairs of the American Nurses' Association.

1 Sep 1983 Col. Connie L. Slewitzke was sworn in as the seventeenth Chief of the Army Nurse Corps. She had been Chief of the Department of Nursing at Letterman Army Medical Center; Chief, 18th Medical Command, Korea; and Assistant Chief of the Army Nurse Corps.

Oct 1983 A bachelor's degree with a major in nursing became a requirement for promotion to the rank of major for all National Guard Army Nurse Corps officers.

Oct 1983 Elements of the 5th MASH and the 307th Medical Battalion, Fort Bragg, North Carolina, deployed to Grenada to support military forces sent to restore stability after the assassination of the nation's leader. Sixteen nurses cared for both military and civilian patients. Six Army nurses received awards for service in Grenada.

Nov 1983 Lt. Col. Nancy Adams joined the newly established Quality Assurance Organization in the Office of the Assistant Secretary of Defense for Health Affairs as Senior Policy Analyst. She served until June 1985.

Nov 1983 The Military Women's Corridor in the Pentagon was dedicated. This permanent exhibit pays tribute to military women for their contributions from the American Revolution to the future.

1984 The expansion of active duty ANC spaces resulted in the assignment of 181 additional ANC officers to new positions within Forces Command (FORSCOM), bringing to 200 the total number of Army nurses based in CONUS field units. Through a memorandum of agreement, these nurses assigned to FORSCOM units were attached to and worked in collocated Health Services Command (HSC) medical treatment facilities (MTFs). Nurses maintained clinical proficiency while being provided opportunities for field nursing–related experiences with their assigned units.

1984 A new concept, Nurse Detachments (NURSEDETS), was formulated to fill critical shortages of operating room nurses (66E) and nurse anesthetists (66F) in USAR medical units. While assigned to existing medical units, nurses were attached elsewhere to separate detachments collocated with Army medical treatment facilities.

1984 ANC officers in the U.S. Army Reserve (USAR) were offered Special Active Duty for Training (SADT) tours to carry out assignments of concern to the USAR. The first officers to orient to the Office of the Chief, Army Nurse Corps, were Col. Julia Paparella, Col. Catherine Foster, Lt. Col. Flora Sullivan, and Maj. Carol Davis.

1984 The Workload Management System for Nursing (WMSN) was developed and implemented. This system was based on a joint effort by the U.S. Army Nurse Corps and the U.S. Navy Nurse Corps. The WMSN is a patient classification system which captures nursing workload based on the patient's severity of illness. Staffing is then based on direct and indirect nursing care requirements. The system recommends the total staffing requirements for a 24-hour period with suggested staffing distribution pattern across the three work shifts.

1984 The Army ROTC Program, which offered nursing scholarships, assumed increasing significance as a source of new Army nurses. In FY 84 accessions through ROTC reached 112. Scholarship cadets are commissioned as second lieutenants and obligated to serve on active duty for four years.

Mar 1984 Maj. Gary Naleski was assigned to the Medical Training Technical Assistance Field Team (TAFT), Taif, Saudi Arabia, in support of the field health services capabilities of the Saudi Arabian Armed Forces (SAAF). Advisory functions entailed providing information, guidance, and assistance in the areas of military doctrine and procedures, development and implementation of instructional programs, training management, and resource allocation. Major Naleski served in Saudi Arabia for eleven months.

Apr 1984 The Army Nurse Corps Fellow Program was established to provide selected ANC officers from local military medical treatment facilities a three-month period of special duty in the Office of the Chief, Army Nurse Corps. The special duty was designed to provide familiarization with the administrative activities essential to the operation of the Office of the Chief, Army Nurse Corps, and to accomplish special projects related to Army nursing, as assigned by the Chief, ANC. The first ANC Fellow was Maj. Dena Norton. The program was later extended to one year. Maj. Kathleen Tracy was the first ANC officer to serve in this assignment for a full year.

Jun 1984 Several former Army Nurse Corps prisoners of war (POWs) from World War II participated in a videotape documentary production, "The Other Side of Freedom," filmed by Department of Defense Audiovisual Agency at the Presidio in San Francisco. Maj. Mary Frank, Army Nurse Corps Historian, served as technical adviser for the documentary, which focused on the experiences of Army nurses in the Philippine Islands in 1941–42 and their subsequent imprisonment for almost three years by the Japanese. The participating veterans were Col. Ruby Bradley, 1st Lt. Helen Nestor, Lt. Col. Madeline Ullom, Lt. Col. Hattie Brantley, Maj. Josephine Nesbit Davis, Capt. Ann Mealer Giles, Capt. Bertha Dworski Henderson, and Capt. Beulah Greenwalt Walcher. Three former POW Navy nurses also appeared in the film. Retitled "We All Came Home: Army and Navy Nurse POWs During World War II," it was released on 26 August 1985.

Jul 1984 The ANC Reserve Components Operating Room Nursing Course was instituted in an effort to alleviate the shortage of operating room nurses in the reserve components. The course was designed in two phases, consisting of eight weeks' didactic and clinical training at Fitzsimons Army Medical Center followed by specific clinical experiences, correspondence courses, seminars, and symposia at the individual's home location. Following Phase II, students returned to Fitzsimons for a comprehensive written and practical examination on operating room nursing.

Aug 1984 The first Army National Guard Chief Nurse Course was held at the Professional Education Center in Arkansas. Fifty-six Chief Nurses from forty-four states and territories attended the course.

Sep 1984 The Brigadier General Lillian Dunlap Endowed Professional Chair in Nursing was dedicated at Incarnate Word College in San Antonio, Texas. General Dunlap was the fourteenth Chief of the Army Nurse Corps.

Oct 1984 The first Nursing Education and Training Preparatory Course for Chiefs of Nursing Education and Training Services was conducted at the Academy of Health Sciences.

1985 Maj. Edith Gunnels was assigned as Senior Program Analyst, Health Promotion and Disease Prevention, a new position with DOD Health Affairs .

Jan 1985 Maj. Carol A. Reineck was the first Army nurse to attend the Armed Forces Staff College (AFSC) in Norfolk, Virginia. She was one of five honor graduates in the class of 285.

Feb 1985 Five Army nurses (four 66H, one 66B) were assigned to the newly opened Fort Drum Health Clinic in support of the 10th Mountain Division Light Infantry.

Mar 1985 Criteria for eligibility for the "A" prefix, awarded by the Surgeon General, expanded to include career specialization in nursing administration, research, and education.

Apr 1985 Capt. Karen Keller was sent to assist the Armed Forces of Liberia (AFL) for 168 days as a member of the Medical Mobile Training Team. The team conducted needs assessments, developed a program of instruction, and conducted training for AFL medical corpsmen.

Sep 1985 Capt. Virginia Koch Bailey, MOS 66E, Fort Ord, California, was the Officer Honor Graduate of her Airborne Training Class at Fort Benning. Of 67 officers who started the course, 55 graduated, including 6 women.

1986 Lt. Col. Shirley Coffey, Nurse Researcher, Department of Virus Diseases, Research and Development Command, served as the first ANC team member within the Retrovirus Group of U.S. Army biomedical scientists. The group's efforts were directed toward the prevention, detection, treatment, and control of Human Immunodeficiency Virus (HIV) and Acquired Immune Deficiency Syndrome (AIDS).

1986 The revised AR 600-85, Alcohol and Drug Abuse Prevention and Control Program (ADAPCP), was published to comply with DOD Directive 1010.14, which required all military services to develop programs to prevent, identify, and treat alcohol and drug impairment among health care professionals.

Oct 1986 Wilcox Army Health Clinic at Fort Drum, New York, became Wilcox U.S. Army Community Hospital. Lt. Col. Patricia LaFond was the first Chief Nurse.

Dec 1986 Brig. Gen. Lillian Dunlap, fourteenth Chief of the Army Nurse Corps, was inducted into the San Antonio Women's Hall of Fame. In 1985 she was appointed to the Governor's Commission for Women in Texas.

Mar 1987 Army medical and nursing personnel served in a humanitarian training mission on the USNS *Mercy*, a Navy hospital ship docked in Subic Bay, Philippines. During this mission, 2d Lt. Ronald Kirkconnell was killed in a helicopter crash while on a training flight.

2 Mar 1987 The lecture hall in the School of Nursing, Incarnate Word College, San Antonio, Texas, was dedicated to the memory of Col. Anna E. Everett, an Army nurse, scholar, and teacher from 1950 to 1976.

May 1987 Lt. Col. Jude O. Larkin was presented the first Colonel Katherine F. Galloway Distinguished Nurse Award. This award, established in 1986, recognizes Army Nurse Corps officers whose contributions merit commendation and contribute to the advancement of nursing practice. Colonel Galloway served as Chief Nurse of the U.S. Army Institute of Surgical Research at Brooke Army Medical Center, Fort Sam Houston, Texas, from 1968 to 1971. She was cited for her exceptional leadership and contributions to the production of medical films and manuscripts regarding nursing care of burns. She also served as Medical-Surgical Supervisor at the 85th Evacuation Hospital and Chief Nurse of the 2d Surgical Hospital in Vietnam.

Jun 1987 Two retired nurses, Lt. Cols. Ernestine Shugart and Cassandra Smith, were the first recipients of the Army Nurse Corps Scholars Fund award at the University of Texas Health Science Center School of Nursing in San Antonio, Texas. The purpose of the award is to honor the professional accomplishments of all ANC retired, reserve, and active duty officers through small research grants. The recipients became known as Scholars of the ANC Fund. Another goal of the Scholars Fund is to establish an ANC Endowed Professorship Chair at the Center.

Jun 1987 Brig. Gen. Lillian Dunlap, the fourteenth Chief of the Army Nurse Corps, received an honorary Doctor of Science degree from Incarnate Word College, San Antonio, Texas. The honorary degree recognizes her significant contributions and leadership to nursing and to the Army Nurse Corps.

Jun 1987 Brig. Gen. Hazel Johnson-Brown, sixteenth Chief of the Army Nurse Corps, received the Alumni Achievement Award in Government from The Catholic University of America.

Jun 1987 First Lt. Elizabeth Ann Jones' death was commemorated twenty years after she was killed in a helicopter crash in Vietnam. Her name, along with

974 others killed in Vietnam, was inscribed on a memorial in Columbia, South Carolina. (See Appendix K.)

Jul 1987 Lt. Col. Charlene Peterson was assigned as the first Chief Nurse of the U.S. ROTC Command. Each of the Cadet Command's four regional headquarters has a Chief Nurse assigned, with nurse counselors assigned throughout the command.

Jul 1987 Lt. Col. William T. Bester was the first Army Nurse Corps officer to serve as the Army Medical Department Regimental Adjutant from July 1987 through June 1988 at Fort Sam Houston, Texas.

1 Sep 1987 Col. Clara Adams-Ender was nominated for promotion to brigadier general and selected to succeed Brig. Gen. Connie L. Slewitzke as Chief of the Army Nurse Corps. Prior to her appointment as Chief, ANC, General Adams-Ender served for three years as Chief, Department of Nursing, Walter Reed Army Medical Center.

22 Oct 1987 A tree was planted on Ohio State University grounds at the site of the Veterans Administration Out-Patient Clinic in honor of Sallie Farmer, a former Army nurse, who was the only surviving female prisoner of war of the World War II era residing in Ohio.

8 Jan 1988 The Smith Well Baby Clinic was dedicated in memory of Capts. Patrick Smith, a Pediatric Nurse Practitioner, and Rosemary Smith, a Community Health Nurse. (See Appendix K.)

Feb 1988 The 8th Evacuation Hospital, Fort Ord, deployed to Fort Hunter Liggett, California, and set up a 400-bed Deployable Medical Systems (DEPMEDS) hospital. Eighty-five Professional Officer Filler System (PROFIS) personnel involved with a paraprofessional staff conducted the DA-directed assessment and validation of the effectiveness of the DEPMEDS and provided Test and Experimentation Command (TEXCOM) with the results. The 8th Evacuation Hospital became the first DEPMEDS hospital as part of the Army's Force Modernization and AMEDD's Medical Force 2000 (MFKK) plan, which focused on standardizing medical facilities throughout the Department of Defense (DOD).

Jan 1989 The 8th Evacuation Hospital conducted the first overseas deployment using the Deployable Medical Systems Hospital to provide patient care in support of the FUERTES CAMINOS 89 road-building project in Honduras. The first surgery and the first live birth occurred in this DEPMEDS facility, as part of the medical Humanitarian Civic Action (HCA) mission. This overseas deployment provided joint training in delivering patient care in a DEPMEDS hospital for the active Army, Army National Guard, and the Army, Navy, and Air Force reserve components.

Jun 1989 Maj. James Keenan, Capt. Andrea Coenen, and Capt. Dennis Driscoll, members of a burn team from the U.S. Army Institute of Surgical Research, were deployed on a mercy mission to the Soviet Union to care for 100 burn patients injured in a gas explosion and train wreck near Ufa, Russia.

Jun 1989 The Army, Navy, and Air Force Chiefs of Nursing testified for the first time together before a Senate subcommittee on defense to address the shortage of professional nurses in the military.

Sep 1989 Lt. Col. Susan McCall deployed with a medical element from the 44th Medical Brigade to St. Croix, Virgin Islands, in support of relief efforts following Hurricane Hugo.

Dec 1989 Army Nurse Corps officers from the 44th Medical Brigade, Fort Bragg, North Carolina, deployed to Panama in support of Operation JUST CAUSE.

May 1990 The Army Nurse Candidate Program was implemented, allowing the Army Nurse Corps to remain competitive with civilian recruiting programs. The program provided candidates a $500 monthly stipend for the last two years of nursing school plus a $5,000 accession bonus to remain on active duty for at least four years.

Aug 1990 Medical operations in support of Operation DESERT SHIELD/DESERT STORM began the second week of August 1990 when the Army Medical Department (AMEDD) received the dual mission of deployment to Southwest Asia and the continuous care of soldiers and their families in the continental United States and overseas. Col. Barbara Smith served as the Army Component, Central Command (ARCENT), Chief Nurse, and Lt. Col. Ruth Cheney served as Chief Nurse of the 44th Medical Brigade.

Sep 1990 Approval of the AMEDD Enlisted Commissioning Program allowed selected enlisted personnel with two years of general education courses to study at an approved college or university nursing program and complete a Baccalaureate of Science in Nursing. Each year, 100 students were to be selected to provide the active component with a steady source of new Army nurses.

The National Defense Authorization Act for 1990–1991 authorized nurse anesthetists special pay bonuses of up to $6,000 per year. It was the first time nurses had been authorized to receive incentive pay.

Dec 1990 The Department of Nursing at Tripler Army Medical Center became the first Army medical center to implement a competency-based orientation, the first to initiate the Accelerated Civilian Nurse Training Program, and the first Army Nursing Department to control all elements of resources. Maj. Donna Patterson was assigned as the project coordinator, as well as serving as Assistant Chief of the Department of Clinical Investigation (DCI).

Jan 1991 By mid-January, medical facilities in support of DESERT SHIELD/DESERT STORM consisted of 44 hospitals: 17 Army Reserve hospitals, 11 National Guard hospitals, and 16 active component hospitals.

Feb 1991 There were over 87,000 AMEDD personnel on active duty during DESERT SHIELD/DESERT STORM, the largest AMEDD deployment since Vietnam. More than 23,000, with 55 percent being from the reserve component, were deployed to Southwest Asia, including 2,265 nurses.

Mar 1991 Col. Jean Reeder served as President of the Association of Operating Room Nurses. She was the first active duty nurse to be elected president of a national nursing organization.

Apr 1991 After graduation from the U.S. Military Academy, West Point, New York, in 1984, 1st Lt. Susan E. Meckfessel was commissioned into the Quartermaster Corps. Following assignments to Germany, the Quartermaster Advanced Course, and Korea, she left active duty to attend nursing school at St. Louis University. On 1 April 1991, Lieutenant Meckfessel was recommissioned into the Army Nurse Corps. She was the first West Point graduate to be appointed into the Army Nurse Corps.

31 May 1991 Brig. Gen. Dorothy B. Pocklington, Individual Mobilization Augmentee (IMA) to the Chief, Army Nurse Corps, for Mobilization and Reserve Affairs, completed her assignment. Col. Marilyn Musachio was promoted to brigadier general and selected as her replacement.

Jun 1991 Maj. Daniel Jergens was the only nurse to accompany the 25th Infantry Division on a humanitarian mission, Operation BALIKATAN, to provide nursing care to displaced Philippine citizens after Mount Pinatubo erupted.

Jul 1991 Lt. Col. Alice L. Demaris was assigned as the Deputy Corps Surgeon for Nursing Activities (DCSNA) for the III Corps, which includes all or part of eight installations: Forts Hood, Carson, Riley, Sill, Polk, Bliss, Sam Houston, and Leavenworth.

Aug 1991 Brig. Gen. Clara Adams-Ender became the first ANC officer to remain on active duty as a general officer after serving as Chief, Army Nurse

Corps. She assumed command of Fort Belvoir, Virginia, and served as Deputy Commanding General, Military District of Washington.

1 Sep 1991 Col. Nancy R. Adams was nominated for promotion to brigadier general and selected to succeed Brig. Gen. Clara L. Adams as nineteenth Chief of the Army Nurse Corps. Prior to her appointment as Chief, General Adams served as Nursing Consultant to the Surgeon General and Chief, Department of Nursing, Frankfurt Army Regional Medical Center.

27 Nov 1991 Col. Nancy R. Adams was promoted to brigadier general and sworn in as the nineteenth Chief of the Army Nurse Corps.

May 1992 The first sixty-five AMEDD Enlisted Commissioning Program (AECP) students were commisioned as ANC officers.

Jun 1992 The Army Nurse Corps began to sponsor a pilot program, the Master's Assistance Program (MAP), through the U.S. Army Recruiting Command to fund, in part, selected new accessions pursuing a Master of Science in Nursing. Also, the Army Nurse Candidate Program (ANCP) and the New Specialized Training Assistance Program (New STRAP) provided financial assistance to individuals in return for service in the Ready Reserve.

Jun 1992 The Colonel Charles J. Reddy Professional Leadership Development Course was instituted to foster the development of leadership skills, knowledge, and behavior in junior Army Nurse Corps officers to prepare them for future leadership roles. The course allows junior officers to meet and work with ANC staff members in key Army leadership positions and to gain an appreciation for the Army Nurse Corps from a wider perspective.

Jul 1992 The Army Nurse Corps Award of Excellence was presented for the first time to a junior ANC officer from each of the three components. The recipients were Capts. Katherine Kelly, active component, Joseph Meegan II, National Guard, and James Morgan, Army Reserve.

Aug 1992 The operating room nurses and anesthetists from the 7th Medical Command (MEDCOM) deployed to Tbilisi, Georgia Republic, and Bishkek, Kirghizstan, to educate local hospital personnel about supplies and equipment donated under the auspices of the humanitarian assistance program.

Aug 1992 Col. Mary T. Sarnecky was selected to research and write the history of the Army Nurse Corps. Colonel Sarnecky was also selected as the first recipient of the New York–Tidewater Chapter's History of Military Medicine Essay Award presented during the annual meeting of the Association of Military Surgeons of the United States in November 1991.

Nov 1992 As part of Operation PROVIDE PROMISE, Army Nurse Corps officers from throughout the 7th MEDCOM deployed to Zagreb, Croatia, to provide health care to the multinational United Nations peacekeeping force.

Dec 1992 Army Community Health Nurses were assigned, on a six-month rotation basis, to the Headquarters Joint Task Force for Brave Medical Element, Honduras.

Jan 1993 Col. Patricia F. Troumbley was selected by the Chief, Army Nurse Corps, as the Army's representative for the first Tri-Service Nursing Research Group (TSNRG).

Jan 1993 Maj. Mary Burman, Chief Nurse of the U.S. Army Medical Research Institute of Infectious Diseases, Fort Detrick, Maryland, was selected as the Honor Graduate in the Air Force's 50th Flight Nurse Course. It was the first course since World War II to include Army nurses.

Jan 1993 The Tri-Service Alcoholism Recovery Department (TRISARD) at the National Naval Medical Center redefined its mission, goals, and objectives. Maj. Melinda Baldridge became the first Army nurse to serve as Chief of TRISARD.

Jan 1993 Army Nurse Corps officers deployed to Somalia to support U.S. troops serving in Operation RESTORE HOPE. The first hospital in Somalia was the 86th Evacuation Hospital which was replaced by the 42d MASH followed by the 46th Combat Support Hospital. This deployment from January 1993 to March 1994 was a humanitarian mission executed under hostile conditions. AMEDD personnel cared for the largest single-day volume of combat casualties since the Vietnam War.

Apr 1993 Two roads by DeWitt Hospital at Fort Belvoir, Virginia, were memorialized as part of the ongoing fiftieth anniversary of World War II. One street was named for Col. Julia C. Stimson, who was superintendent of the ANC from 1919 to 1937, and the other street was named after Pvt. Frank J. Petrarca, a medic during World War II.

Jun 1993 Maj. Reymundo Lariosa was assigned for six months to El Salvador as the only nurse of a humanitarian medical treatment team. He provided nursing care, assisted with training Salvadoran medics, and evaluated health needs within garrison areas. In addition, he served as a nursing consultant to the El Salvador medical forces.

Aug 1993 Brig. Gen. Clara Adams-Ender retired after thirty-three years of military service. After serving as the eighteenth Chief of the Army Nurse Corps, General Adams-Ender served for two years as Commanding General, United

States Army, Fort Belvoir, as well as Deputy Commanding General, United States Army Military District of Washington, Fort Belvoir, Virginia.

Oct 1993 Brig. Gen. Nancy Adams, Chief of the Army Nurse Corps, was appointed Assistant Surgeon General as well as the Director of Personnel for the Surgeon General.

Oct 1993 The U.S. Army Medical Command (MEDCOM) Provisional was activated in San Antonio, Texas.

23 Oct 1993 Col. Mildred Irene Clark, twelfth Chief of the Army Nurse Corps, was inducted into the Michigan Women's Hall of Fame.

11 Nov 1993 The Vietnam Women's Memorial was dedicated in the nation's capital. The memorial honors the women who served during the Vietnam era. (See Appendix K.)

Dec 1993 The 212th MASH deployed to Zagreb in support of the United Nations forces in Croatia with Operation PROVIDE PROMISE.

Dec 1993 Lt. Col. Mozettia Henley and Capt. Rebecca LaChance were selected to attend the Medical Research Fellowship program at Walter Reed Army Institute of Research. This was the first year in which individuals other than physicians were allowed to compete.

Mar 1994 The Regional Nursing Research Coordinator role was created to decentralize the nursing research structure, using a regional concept with the Nursing Research Advisory Board as the managing body.

Jun 1994 The Harriet H. Werley Chair in Nursing Research was established in honor of Colonel Werley (Ret.) at the College of Nursing, University of Illinois, Chicago.

Jun 1994 Jesse Brown, Secretary, Department of Veterans Affairs (VA), appointed three retired Army nurses, Brig Gens. Connie Slewitzke and Clara Adams-Ender and Col. Lois Johns, to the VA Advisory Committee on Women Veterans. They will serve until 1997 and provide advice, consultation, and reports to the Secretary regarding programs for women veterans.

Aug 1994 Col. Theora Mitchell became the first ANC officer to attend the Wharton Nurse Fellows program, a three-week business management program underwritten by Johnson & Johnson and conducted at the University of Pennsylvania's Wharton School of Business.

2 Aug 1994 Brig. Gen. Nancy Adams, Chief of the Army Nurse Corps, was selected as Commander, United States Army Center for Health Promotion and Preventive Medicine (CHPPM). The focus of this new command is to support health promotion, public health, and preventive medicine throughout the Army.

Oct 1994 Maj. Nelly Aleman-Guzman was presented the Purple Heart for injuries received in 1989 while serving in El Salvador. She was the first female active duty Army nurse to receive the award since the Vietnam era.

2 Oct 1994 Health Services Command (HSC) was deactivated, and the U.S. Army Medical Command (MEDCOM) lost provisional status, becoming a fully activated command.

Jan 1995 Capt. Bethany Alexander became the first nurse to compete and be selected for command of an AMEDD Center and School training company. She commanded Company D, 232d Medical Battalion.

Jul 1995 The Assistant Chief of the Army Nurse Corps will serve with the Army Staff (ARSTAF) as the Assistant to the Surgeon General for Nursing, being the primary staff officer at the corporate level for all Army nursing operations.

Appendix A

SUPERINTENDENTS AND CHIEFS OF THE ARMY NURSE CORPS

Dita H. Kinney	15 Mar 1901–31 Jul 1909
Jane A. Delano	12 Aug 1909–31 Mar 1912
Isabel McIsaac	1 Apr 1912–21 Sep 1914
Dora E. Thompson	22 Sep 1914–29 Dec 1919
	*Major**
Julia C. Stimson	30 Dec 1919–31 May 1937
Julia O. Flikke	1 Jun 1937–13 Mar 1942
	Colonel
Julia O. Flikke	13 Mar 1942–30 Jun 1943
Florence A. Blanchfield	1 Jul 1943–30 Sep 1947
Mary G. Phillips	1 Oct 1947–30 Sep 1951
Ruby F. Bryant	1 Oct 1951–30 Sep 1955
Inez Haynes	1 Oct 1955–31 Aug 1959
Margaret Harper	1 Sep 1959–31 Aug 1963
Mildred Irene Clark	1 Sep 1963–21 Aug 1967
Anna Mae Hays	1 Sep 1967–10 Jun 1970
	Brigadier General
Anna Mae Hays	11 Jun 1970–31 Aug 1971
Lillian Dunlap	1 Sep 1971–31 Aug 1975
Madelyn N. Parks	1 Sep 1975–31 Aug 1979
Hazel W. Johnson	1 Sep 1979–31 Aug 1983
Connie L. Slewitzke	1 Sep 1983–31 Aug 1987
Clara L. Adams-Ender	1 Sep 1987–31 Aug 1991
Nancy R. Adams	27 Nov 1991–

*Relative Rank (See entry for 4 June 1920)

Appendix B

FIRST ASSISTANTS TO THE SUPERINTENDENTS*
AND ASSISTANT CHIEFS
OF THE
ARMY NURSE CORPS

Edith A. Mury First Executive Assistant Assistant Superintendent (Sep 1918)	Nov 1917–Mid-1919
Julia C. Stimson Assistant Superintendent and Acting Superintendent	20 Jul 1919–30 Dec 1919
Sayres L. Milliken CPT	Late 1919–Oct 1935
Nena Shelton CPT	Nov 1935–Jan 1939
Florence A. Blanchfield CPT/LTC	Feb 1939–Jan 1943
Acting Superintendent	10 Feb 1943–Jun 1943
Mary G. Phillips MAJ/LTC	15 May 1943–Jul 1945
Margaret E. Aaron LTC	Sep 1945–Nov 1946
Mary G. Phillips LTC	Mar 1947–13 Aug 1947
Acting Superintendent	14 Aug 1947–30 Sep 1947
Katharine E. Baltz (Hayes) LTC	Oct 1947–Aug 1951

*Title used to avoid confusion with the statutory grade of "Assistant Superintendent" from July 1918–April 1947 (relative rank of captain to December 1942 and captain to lieutenant colonel thereafter)

Rosalie D. Calhoun LTC	Sep 1951–Aug 1955
Margaret Harper MAJ/LTC	Sep 1955–Aug 1959
Harriet A. Dawley (Wells) MAJ/LTC	Sep 1959–Jul 1963
Anna Mae Hays LTC	1 Sep 1963–31 Aug 1966
Gladys E. Johnson LTC/COL	1 Sep 1966–30 Sep 1967
Nelly Newell COL	1 Oct 1967–31 May 1970
Louise C. Rosasco COL	1 Jun 1970–31 Dec 1971
Edith J. Bonnet COL	1 Jan 1972–31 Jan 1973
Rose V. Straley COL	1 Feb 1973–31 Aug 1974
Edith M. Nuttall COL	1 Sep 1974–30 Apr 1978
Virginia L. Brown COL	1 May 1978–31 May 1980
Connie L. Slewitzke COL	1 Jun 1980–31 Aug 1983
Eily P. Gorman COL	28 Sep 1983–29 Sep 1987
John M. Hudock COL	1 Oct 1987–29 Sep 1991
Terris E. Kennedy COL	1 Sep 1991–

Appendix C

DR. ANITA NEWCOMB MCGEE AWARD

The Anita Newcomb McGee Award of the National Society, Daughters of the American Revolution (DAR), honors the memory of Dr. McGee, who organized the Army Nurse Corps during the Spanish-American War. The award is sponsored yearly by the DAR to an active duty Nurse Corps officer, with the grade of captain or above and in a career status, selected by the Surgeon General as the "U.S. Army Nurse of the Year."

1967	CPT Linda A. Bowman
1968	LTC Sara Lundy
1969	CPT Josephine A. Goligoski
1970	LT Sharon Ann Lane
1971	BG Anna Mae Hays
1972	COL Hazel W. Johnson
1973	COL Drusilla Poole
1974	COL Nellie M. Hill
1975	COL Mary Mulqueen
1976	COL Marjorie J. Wilson
1977	COL Mary Jane Carr
1978	COL Edith M. Nuttall
1979	COL Patricia M. Miller
1980	COL Virginia L. Brown
1981	LTC Naldean Borg
1982	LTC Janet R. Southby

1983	LTC Joyce Johnson-Bowles LTC Susie Sherrod
1984	LTC James D. Vail
1985	MAJ Jayne O'Donnell
1986	LTC Nancy C. Molter
1987	LTC Barbara S. Turner
1988	LTC Diane K. Corcoran
1989	LTC Frannie M. Rettig
1990	LTC Bonnie L. Jennings
1991	LTC Kathryn B. Scheidt
1992	LTC Carol A. Reineck
1993	LTC Jane Y. Yaws
1994	COL Irene M. Rich
1995	LTC Cynthia A. Abbott

Appendix D

BOVARD AWARD

The Evangeline G. Bovard Award honors the Letterman Army Medical Center's outstanding Army nurse each year. The late Col. Robert Skelton established the award in 1956 in tribute to his first wife, who was an Army nurse. Evangeline Bovard's first duty station was Letterman, and she passed away in 1955 at Letterman. With the inactivation of Letterman Army Hospital, the award was transferred to Madigan Medical Center in December 1993. (See Appendix K.)

1957	CPT Lenora B. Weirick
1958	MAJ Ruth Edenfield
1959	MAJ Iola R. McClellan CPT Teresa M. Brown
1960	MAJ Hendrina Jankowski
1961	1LT Carmelita P. Clukey 1LT Mary K. LaVigne
1962	MAJ Helen E. Grant
1963	MAJ Irene G. R. Zieske
1964	CPT Hazel W. Johnson
1965	MAJ Mary Rita
1966	LTC Margaret C. Stafford
1967	LTC Marjorie J. Conly
1968	MAJ Elizabeth E. Campbell
1969	LTC Romona E. DeLaney
1970	MAJ Oswald A. Ferry CPT Eileen J. Gentile
1971	CPT Loretta Forlaw
1972	LTC Marie L. Rodgers
1973	CPT Erie D. Capps

1974 CPT Larry W. Weigum

1975 LTC Doris H. Ledbetter

1976 CPT Marie T. Sweet

1977 MAJ Kathleen Shafer

1978 CPT Kathleen M. Scanlan

1979 CPT Dena A. Norton

1980 MAJ Kenneth Gunnell

1981 CPT Shirley Jackson

1982 CPT Patrick M. Garvin

1983 CPT Patricia L. O'Rourke

1984 MAJ Linda Crouch

1985 MAJ Harriet Scheele

1986 LTC Joyce G. Shank

1987 LTC Karen A. Waxdahl

1988 MAJ Carol A. Flynn

1989 MAJ Rebecca Loomis
1LT Patricia Shelly

1990 MAJ Analiza Savage
CPT Angela Martinelli

1991 LTC Susan Spaulding
CPT Mona Bingham

1992 MAJ Sarah M. Nordquist
CPT Joe D. Pena
CPT Adoracion G. Soria

1994 MAJ Stacy Young-McCaughan
1LT Laura Moergeli

1995 MAJ Joan Campanaro
CPT Jacqueline Parker

Appendix E

FELLOWS OF THE AMERICAN ACADEMY OF NURSING

The American Academy of Nursing is an independent organization under the sponsorship of the American Nurses' Association and is an active working body of nursing leaders and scholars in education, practice, administration, and research. Fellows are elected to membership based on their contributions to the nursing profession.

1973	LTC Geraldene Felton (Ret.) LTC Phyllis J. Verhonick (Ret.) LTC Harriet Werley (Ret.)
1974	COL Rosemary T. McCarthy (Ret.) COL Lois Johns (Ret.)
1981	COL Ira Gunn (Ret.)
1984	BG Hazel Johnson-Brown (Ret.) LTC Terry Misener (Ret.)
1988	COL Barbara Turner (Ret.) COL Cecil Drain (Ret.)
1990	BG Clara Adams-Ender (Ret.) COL Mary Frank (Ret.) BG Dorothy Pocklington (Ret.)
1991	COL Bonnie Jennings
1992	COL Jean Reeder
1993	BG Lillian Dunlap (Ret.) (Honorary) BG Nancy Adams
1994	COL Claudia Bartz

Appendix F

THE PHYLLIS J. VERHONICK AWARD

The award is presented to an active duty, reserve, or National Guard Army nurse who demonstrates excellence in research that significantly contributes to nursing and improves patient care outcomes.

1981	MAJ Susie Sherrod
1982	CPT Loretta Garcia, USAR
1984	MAJ Adele Rehm
1986	MAJ Irene Rich
1988	LTC Ruth Rea MAJ Regina Girlando
1990	MAJ Linda Yoder MAJ Janet R. Harris
1992	MAJ Linda Yoder CPT Bruce Schoneboom
1994	COL Cynthia Gurney LTC Gail McClellan MAJ Elizabeth Mittelstaedt MAJ Stacey Young-McCaughan

Appendix G

ARMY NURSE CORPS WHITE HOUSE MEDICAL UNIT

1979–82	CPT Vicky Sheldon
1982–87	MAJ Dianne Capps
1984–87	CPT Ann Treleven
1987–89	MAJ Barbara Eller
1987–93	LTC Paula Trivett
1989–93	MAJ Arthur Wallace
1993–95	MAJ Leana Fox-Johnson
1993–95	CPT Maureen Donohue

Appendix H

ARMY NURSE CORPS MEDAL
LEADERSHIP - SCHOLARSHIP - PARTICIPATION

The Army Nurse Corps Medal is an award presented to the outstanding Army Nurse Corps officer upon completion of the resident AMEDD Officer Advanced Course. The medal was presented for the first time in 1961 and is given twice a year.

Jun 61	CPT Angela Hennek
Dec 61	CPT Corrinne Sater
Jun 62	CPT Sally Stallard
Dec 62	CPT Linda Lee
Jun 63	CPT John Robinson
Dec 63	MAJ Marthanne Kingsley
Jun 64	CPT John Girvan
Dec 64	CPT Anthony Soltys
Jun 65	CPT Frances Hiers
Dec 65	1LT Amelia Carson
Jun 66	MAJ Mary Condit
Dec 66	CPT Jean Johnson
Jun 67	MAJ Rose Munchbach
Dec 67	CPT Charles L. Matteson
Feb 68	CPT Nickey J. McCasland
Jun 68	CPT Felicitus E. Ferington
Dec 68	CPT Martha S. Johnson
Mar 69	CPT Joan R. Groce
Jun 69	MAJ Claire M. McQuail
Dec 69	CPT John A. Danner

Jun 70	CPT Janice M. Nelson
Dec 70	CPT Patricia J. Basta
Jun 71	CPT Franklin L. Metcalf
Dec 71	CPT David H Zuelke
Jun 72	CPT Kay F. Layman
Dec 72	CPT Evelyn E. Boaz
Jun 73	CPT Jude O. Larkin
Dec 73	CPT Clement J. Markarian
Jun 74	CPT Mary C. Flinchbaugh
Dec 74	CPT Eda L. Weiskotten
Jun 75	CPT Linda C. Antle
Dec 75	CPT Sandra L. Hamper
Jun 76	CPT Patricia A. Warren
Dec 76	MAJ Elizabeth G. Ryan
Jun 77	CPT Karen S. Haase
Dec 77	CPT Margaret J. Zweig
Jun 78	CPT Donna Sylvester
Dec 78	MAJ Lawrence A. Hamer CPT Timothy P. Williams
Jun 79	CPT Ruth Rae
Dec 79	CPT Mary Jo Heger
Jun 80	CPT Colleen D. Blazier
Dec 80	CPT Mary E. Gaskill
Jun 81	CPT Catherine B. Hilliard
Dec 81	CPT Linda S. Chancey
Jun 82	CPT Pamela J. Hildreath CPT Patricia F. Prather

Dec 82	CPT Martha E. Brown
Jun 83	CPT Annette E. Etnyre
Dec 83	CPT Pamela K. Bailey
Jun 84	CPT Elaine M. DeCesare
Dec 84	CPT Patricia Saulsbery
May 85	CPT Amy M. Ertter
Dec 85	CPT Patricia O'Rourke
May 86	MAJ Mary Bradshaw
Dec 86	CPT Michael Burton
May 87	CPT Holly Davis
Dec 87	CPT Susan West
Feb 88	CPT Laura Ruse
May 88	CPT Kathryn Dotter
Dec 88	CPT Michael McCarthy
Feb 89	CPT Sharon Steele
May 89	CPT John Blower
Dec 89	CPT Faith Kline
May 90	CPT Peggy Iverson
Dec 90	CPT Katherine Hightower
May 91	CPT Suzanne Pieklik
Dec 91	CPT Shawn Kueter
Dec 92	CPT Kimberly A. Smith
Jun 93	CPT Jean Boyle
Jun 94	MAJ Nancy Soltez
Dec 94	CPT Patricia Hall
May 95	CPT John Canady

Appendix J

AMITA AWARD

The American Italian Awards, Incorporated (AMITA), presents twelve awards annually in New York City to honor American women of Italian descent who have distinguished themselves in their chosen field. The award has not been presented since the mid-1980s.

1962	CPT Teresa J. Tauroney
1963	MAJ Maria L. La Conte
1964	LTC Katherine R. Jump
1965	LTC Josephine M. Ognibene
1966	COL Louise Rosasco
1967	MAJ Doris M. Calcagni
1968	COL Ruth Pacini Satterfield
1970	LTC Mary Rita
1971	LTC Anna E. Antonicci
1972	LTC Marian Barbieri
1973	LTC Philomina M. Tardio
1975	LTC Anna Frederico BG Madelyn N. Parks
1976	LTC Marguarite J. Rossi
1977	LTC Mary Lou Spine
1981	COL Eugenia A. Vineys

Appendix K

MEMORIALS

1902 A monument to Spanish-American War nurses who gave their lives in 1898 was dedicated on 22 May 1902 in the nurses' section of Arlington National Cemetery. The memorial was given by surviving Spanish-American War nurses who paid tribute "To Our Comrades."

1906 The state of Illinois erected a statue in a park in Galesburg, Illinois, honoring Mary Ann Bickerdyke, a Sanitary Commission worker in the West who ministered to the needs of the wounded in no less than nineteen battles. An inscription on the monument reads:

"Mother Bickerdyke (1861–Army Nurse–1865)
She Outranks Me. —General Sherman."

1914 A large bronze statue, "a tribute of honor and gratitude" to Civil War nurses, was erected in the rotunda of the State Capitol Building, Boston, Massachusetts, by the Massachusetts Daughters of Veterans organization. The statue depicts a woman caring for a wounded Union Army soldier. The inscription on the base of the statue reads: "To the Army Nurses from 1861 to 1865, Angels of Mercy and Life Amid Scenes of Conflict and Death."

1915 The cornerstone of a memorial building honoring the heroic women of the Civil War was laid on 27 March 1915 in Washington, D.C. The building, dedicated on 12 May 1917 and given as headquarters to the American National Red Cross in perpetuity, was to commemorate the women of both the North and the South who "braved the discomforts of fever-striken camp or crowded ward to lessen the suffering of the sick and wounded."

1917 The McIsaac Loan Fund was established in memory of Isabel McIsaac, third Superintendent of the Army Nurse Corps. Loans from the fund were made available to nurses to further their education.

1918 The first scholarship in the Washington University School of Nursing, St. Louis, Missouri, was awarded. The scholarship, named for Julia C. Stimson who had gone to France in May 1917 as Chief Nurse of Base Hospital No. 21, was funded by the interest from $4 million given by an anonymous donor. The scholarship was to be used by graduates of the Washington University School of Nursing for advanced preparation for teaching, administration, and public health positions.

1919 A flag with a single blue star, representing 19,877 Red Cross nurses who had been on active duty with the Army Nurse Corps and Navy Nurse Corps and the American Red Cross in overseas areas, and 198 gold stars, representing nurses who died during World War I, was placed in the National Headquarters Building, American Red Cross, Washington, D.C

1919 The Jane A Delano Post Number 6, Washington Department of the District of Columbia, American Legion, was chartered on 9 July 1919. The post, composed only of nurses, was established as a living memorial to the second Superintendent of the Army Nurse Corps, Jane A. Delano. Another American Legion Post, the Helen Fairchild Nurses Post 412, in Philadelphia, Pennsylvania, was named for an Army Reserve nurse who died in France during World War I.

1920 A scholarship fund for the education of nurses for tuberculosis work was established by the Alabama State Nurses' Association as a memorial to Alabama nurses who died in the service during World War I. In 1925, the purpose of the fund was changed to further the education of public health nurses.

1922 The nurses' residence at Harper Hospital, Detroit, Michigan, erected under the auspices of Senator James Couzens as a memorial to the Harper Hospital nurses who had served in World War I, was named the Emily A McLaughlin Hall. Miss McLaughlin served as a contract nurse in the Spanish-American War at the Presidio Hospital, San Francisco, and received several awards for her services as Chief Nurse, Base Hospital No. 17, Dijon, France, during World War I.

1923 Four memorial tablets were placed in memory of the officers, nurses, and enlisted men of the Medical Department of the Army who lost their lives during World War I. The tablets were placed in the Army Medical School at the Army Medical Center in Washington, D.C. (later Walter Reed Army Institute of Research, Walter Reed Army Medical Center); Letterman General Hospital, San Francisco; Fitzsimons General Hospital, Denver, Colorado; and at the Army Field Medical School, Carlisle Barracks, Pennsylvania.

1924 The "Nuns of the Battlefield" memorial was dedicated on 20 September 1924 in honor of the members of religious orders who had been employed by the Union Army to care for sick and wounded military men during the Civil War. The monument, located in a park in the District of Columbia, consisted of a granite shaft with a large bronze panel portraying twelve nuns representing various religious groups who served in Army hospitals. The monument was sponsored by the Ladies Auxiliary of the Ancient Order of Hibernians in America.

1927 The names of 101 Army and Army Reserve nurses who died during World War I were placed under a representation of the Army Nurse Corps insignia in the Cloister at the American Pro-Cathedral Church of the Holy Trinity, Paris, France. The names of the Army Nurse Corps members were placed in the third bay of the cloister alongside remembrances to men of American combat divisions.

A figure of an American nurse in a blue service uniform with a crimson-lined cape was placed in the Pantheon de la Guerre, Paris, France. The figure, placed among scenes depicting events of World War I, was representative of nurses from the United States Army and Navy and the American Red Cross who served overseas during World War I.

The names of ten Regular Army nurses and ninety-one reserve nurses, Nurse Corps, U.S. Army, who died while serving with the American Expeditionary Forces, were placed in the Livre d'Or (Book of Gold) which was deposited in the archives of the city of Rheims, France.

1928 The cornerstone of the World War Memorial was laid on 31 May 1928. The building was dedicated to "the Heroic American Women in the World War." This memorial building was intended for use by the District of Columbia Chapter of the American Red Cross. Twenty-one organizations of women who were active in war work, including the nursing services of the Army and the Navy, participated in laying mortar upon the stone. The building was dedicated on 19 March 1930. The first column at the left of the north entrance was dedicated to nursing and inscribed "To Jane A. Delano and the 296 Nurses Who Lost Their Lives in the War."

1929 A statue representing an Army nurse was added to the monument in honor of America's World War dead located in a plot maintained by an American Legion Post in Woodlawn Park Cemetery, Miami, Florida. The four figures completing the memorial represented the Army, the Navy, the Marine Corps, and the Army Nurse Corps.

1930 A monument, the gift of Col. Frank McDermott of Seattle, Washington, honoring the men of the 91st Division, American Expeditionary Forces, World War I, was dedicated at Fort Lewis, Washington. Among the figures on the memorial was a large statue of an Army Reserve nurse caring for a wounded soldier.

1931 The Memorial Chapel, Walter Reed Army Medical Center, Washington, D.C., was dedicated on 21 May 1931 as "A Memorial to the Men Who Gave Their Lives to Service." In the chapel, the first window on the west side was placed as a memorial to the 205 members of the Army Nurse Corps who died in active service during World War I between 6 April 1917 and 11 November 1918. The window, donated by the Corps and presented by Maj. Julia C. Stimson, Superintendent of the Army Nurse Corps, had as its distinctive marks the Lamp of Knowledge and the Caduceus and bore the words "In Memory of the Army Nurse Corps."

1931 L'Ecole Florence Nightingale (Florence Nightingale School) was dedicated on 25 June 1931 in Bordeaux, France, as a memorial to American nurses who died in service during World War I. Funding for the school building and for dormitories of the school of nursing was begun in 1920 by American nurses as a tribute to their comrades. An American Nurses Memorial Medal was struck on the occasion of the laying of the cornerstone of the school.

1931 The District of Columbia War Memorial, located in Potomac Park, Washington, D.C., was dedicated on Armistice Day in honor of the men and women of the armed forces from the District who served in World War I. The memorial, a circular marble bandstand of Doric-type architecture, bore the names of District military personnel, including Army and Army Reserve nurses, who died during World War I.

1934 The Jane A. Delano Memorial, a bronze statue depicting "The Spirit of Nursing," was dedicated on 26 April to Jane A. Delano and 296 nurses of the Army, the Navy, and the Red Cross who died in World War I, 1914–1918. The statue was placed in a square in downtown Washington, D.C., surrounded on three sides by the white marble buildings of the American Red Cross.

1942 On 15 November, a nurses' recreation hall at Fort McClellan, Alabama, was dedicated to Julia Lide, an Army nurse who served in the Spanish-American War and World War I. Miss Lide had been cited by the Commanding General, 3d Division, in France during World War I for extraordinary performance of duty under fire at Chateau Thierry, France, and had been awarded the Croix de Guerre by the French government. Miss Lide died at Base Hospital No. 17 in France on 24 February 1919.

1943 On 1 July, nurses' quarters constructed at Finney General Hospital, Thomasville, Georgia, were dedicated to the memory of 2d Lt. Lillie Ozelle Wages. Lieutenant Wages was killed in an automobile accident on her way from Camp Blanding, Florida, to a new assignment at St. Petersburg, Florida. District 2, Georgia State Nurses' Association, placed the memorial tablet honoring Lieutenant Wages.

1944 Seven nurses' quarters at Finney General Hospital, Thomasville, Georgia, were named in honor of thirty-five Army nurses who were left on Bataan shortly after the United States entered World War II. Each of the seven quarters was furnished a plaque with the names of five of the Army nurses.

The dining hall was dedicated to thirty-one other nurses who served at Corregidor and were left in the Philippine Islands as prisoners of war. (All of the Army nurses were subsequently rescued or later liberated from Santo Tomas Internment Camp. See chronology entries for 9 April 1942 and 6 May 1942.)

1944 On 24 May, a hospital ship was named *The Emily H. M. Weder* in honor of Major Weder, who entered the Army Nurse Corps in 1918 and died at Walter Reed General Hospital in 1943. Major Weder had been chief operating room nurse at Letterman General Hospital and Walter Reed General Hospital.

1944 On 29 May, a hospital ship was named *The Blanche F. Sigman* in honor of Lieutenant Sigman and her colleagues, 1st Lt. Carrie Sheetz and 2d Lt. Marjorie G. Morrow, who were killed when the 95th Evacuation Hospital at Anzio was bombed during World War II.

1944 On 11 December, the U.S. Army's twenty-first hospital ship was named *The Ernestine A. Koranda* in honor of Lieutenant Koranda, ANC, who died in an airplane crash on 19 December 1943 in the Southwest Pacific.

1945 The Women's Club of Dallas County, Alabama, purchased a bomber aircraft for use by the U.S. Army Air Corps, to be named the *Kitty Driskell Barber* in honor of an Army nurse who was killed when the plane in which she was flying went down in the Mediterranean.

1945 On 13 February, the U.S. Army's hospital ship with the largest patient capacity (1,628 patients) was named *The Frances Y. Slanger* in honor of Lieutenant Slanger who was killed 21 October 1944 when struck by a German shell in her tented hospital area.

1945 On 13 February, a hospital ship was named *The Aleda E. Lutz* in honor of Lieutenant Lutz, ANC, who was killed on a flying mission to evacuate wounded personnel from forward areas. Lieutenant Lutz had flown more than 190 evacuation missions and had been awarded the Air Medal with four Oak Leaf Clusters. The Distinguished Flying Cross was awarded posthumously.

1947 The burial site of 2d Lt. Louise W. Bosworth, ANC, in Hamm, Luxembourg, was adopted by the National Association of Nurses in Luxembourg "as a sign of gratitude to those who died in order to give us back our freedom." Bosworth died while serving with the 12th Evacuation Hospital in Luxembourg during World War II.

1948 A library at Boston City Hospital, Boston, Massachusetts, was named the Morse-Slanger Library in honor of two graduates of the school of nursing who lost their lives while serving as Army nurses during World War II. The nurses were 2d Lt. Frances Slanger and 2d Lt. Dorothy Morse. Portraits of both nurses, provided by their classmates, were hung in the library.

1951 In celebration of the centennial of Anna C. Maxwell's birth, a fellowship providing full tuition and university fees for one year of study in nursing at Teachers College, Division of Nursing Education, Columbia University, including meals and lodging, was established. The fellowship honored Miss Maxwell, a contract nurse in the Spanish-American War. The first fellowship was awarded to Frances Sara Beck of London. A total of three fellowships were awarded from 1952–1956.

1956 A "Works of Mercy" window, installed in the Cathedral of St. John the Divine, New York, New York, was dedicated to the American nurses who had given their lives in the service of their country and, more specifically, to the nurses from St. Luke's Hospital School of Nursing who served with the armed forces during both world wars. The service of the nurses was represented by the Badge of France and the Badge of England, placed on either side of the St. Luke's Hospital seal.

1957 The Congress of the United States unanimously voted to recognize the Altar of the Nation at the Cathedral of the Pines in Rindge, New Hampshire, originally established in 1945 as a memorial to all American war dead. In 1967, the Memorial Bell Tower of the cathedral was dedicated as a national memorial for all American women who sacrificed their lives for their country. A bronze tablet on the north arch of the tower depicts Clara Barton, founder of the American Red Cross, assisting a wounded soldier from the battlefield during the Civil War. This plaque honors the women nurses serving the combat forces.

1962 The Marjorie Gertrude Morrow Memorial Library at the Iowa Methodist School of Nursing was named in honor of 2d Lt. Marjorie Morrow, ANC, who was one of three nurses of the 95th Evacuation Hospital killed during a bombing raid on Anzio beachhead in Italy on 7 February 1944.

1965 A commemorative chair plaque engraved "Anna C. Maxwell, RN" was dedicated with the opening of the new auditorium of the College of Physicians and Surgeons, Columbia University. Situated on the back of seat 18, Row L, located in the orchestra, it honors Ms. Maxwell, a Spanish-American War contract nurse.

1966 The Captain Catherine Weadock Newell Center, the former School of Nursing at St. Mary's Hospital, Tucson, Arizona, was renamed in honor of an alumna who had joined the Army Nurse Corps during World War II. Captain Newell served with distinction in Europe and later in Japan. Captain Newell died at Walter Reed General Hospital in 1954.

1967 A fifty-star American flag, presented to the Brookline, Massachusetts, American Legion Post No. 11 by three students in the Army Student Nurse Program, was used thereafter as the flag to be flown over the post in honor and memory of Army nurses.

1968 The Lane County Chapter, American National Red Cross, Eugene, Oregon, dedicated its Board of Directors' Room to the memory of Maj. Maude C. Davison, Army Nurse Corps, who served with great distinction from World War I through World War II. After the fall of Bataan on 6 May 1942, Captain Davison was taken prisoner of war by the Japanese and served as the Principal Chief Nurse in charge of the nursing staff at Santo Tomas Internment Camp, Manila, P.I., until after the liberation when she was relieved by Army nurses who arrived on 9 February 1945. She was the recipient of no less than twelve awards, including the Bronze Star Medal and the Legion of Merit. Major Davison retired on 31 January 1946. She was born on 27 March 1885 in Cannington, Ontario, Canada; she died on 11 June 1956 in Long Beach, California.

1973 A life-size statue of 1st Lt. Sharon A. Lane, Army Nurse Corps, was unveiled at Aultman Hospital, Canton, Ohio. Lieutenant Lane was a 1965 graduate of the Aultman Hospital School of Nursing. The only Army Nurse

Corps officer to be killed as a result of enemy action during the Vietnam War, Lieutenant Lane was fatally wounded on 8 June 1969 during an enemy rocket attack while she was on duty at the 312th Evacuation Hospital in Chu Lai, Republic of Vietnam. The base of the bronze statue carries the inscription, "Born to Honor, Ever at Peace," and the names of 110 local servicemen who died in Vietnam.

1978 The Julia Lide Monument Circle, located at Fort McClellan, Alabama, in front of Noble Army Community Hospital at Fort McClellan, Alabama, was dedicated. Julia Lide was the only Alabama nurse who died during World War I while serving with the Army Nurse Corps. During the war she was cited by Col. David L. Stone, the commanding officer of the 3d Division, American Expeditionary Forces in Europe, for "extraordinary performance of duty, while under fire at Chateau Thierry, France."

1984 The Vietnam Memorial, located in Washington, D.C., bears the names of nine Army nurses who died while serving in Vietnam.

1984 The Vietnam Women's Memorial Project, Inc., was organized for the purpose of creating a monument for the women who served in Vietnam. The statue was to represent and honor all women who served during the Vietnam War, from every branch of military service as well as from other private and governmental agencies.

1986 The life-size bronze stone statue at the North Carolina Vietnam Veterans Memorial was dedicated in the fall of 1986 and placed on Union Square in Raleigh, North Carolina. This memorial reminds all who view it of the enduring value of a common effort, among people of different backgrounds, toward a common goal.

11 Nov 1987 The first military nurses' memorial monument in the state of Massachusetts honoring military nurses throughout history was dedicated in North Weymouth, Massachusetts. Six lines from the poem "Where the Soldier Was" by Col. Maude Smith (Ret.) are inscribed on the stone.

Jan 1988 The Smith Well Baby Clinic at Colonel Florence A. Blanchfield Army Community Hospital, Fort Campbell, Kentucky, was dedicated in memory of Capt. Patrick Smith, a Pediatric Nurse Practitioner, and Capt. Rosemary Smith, a Community Health Nurse. This clinic and a scholarship for nursing students at Austin Peay State University serve to commemorate the Smiths following their tragic deaths in their home in 1987.

20 Jun 1989 A road at Fort Belvoir, Virginia, was dedicated in memory of Lt. Sharon Lane, who died in June 1969, the only American servicewoman killed by direct enemy fire in Vietnam. Sharon Lane Road is the first road at Fort Belvoir named for a Vietnam veteran and the first named for a woman. She received the Bronze Star with a "V" for Valor, the Gallantry Cross with Palm, the Purple Heart, and National Defense and Vietnam Service Medals.

Her name is listed on Panel 23W, line 112, of the Vietnam Veterans' Memorial in Washington, D.C.

Jul 1989 The AMEDD Museum was officially opened after the dedication ceremony on 24 July 1989 in San Antonio, Texas. The new museum has 16,770 square feet of space, including a large exhibit hall, a skylit gallery, a library, and a lecture hall. A planned phase II expansion will add another exhibit hall and pavilion.

June 1991 Fitzsimons Army Medical Center officially changed the name of the street leading from the south gate to the hospital to Sharon A. Lane Drive in memory of Lieutenant Lane.

11 Nov 1993 The Vietnam Women's Memorial bronze sculpture of three military women (one tending a wounded soldier, another standing with a hand on the shoulder of the first and gazing skyward as if looking for the "Dust-Off" helicopter, and the third kneeling behind the other two) was dedicated in Washington, D.C.

Dec 1993 A new facility at the Wisconsin veterans home was named in memory of 2d Lt. Ellen Ainsworth who was killed in action in World War II.

Dec 1993 With the inactivation of Letterman Army Hospital, Presidio of San Francisco, William Bovard, nephew of Evangeline Bovard, requested that the Army Nurse of the Year (Bovard) Award be transferred to either Fort Huachuca, where Evangeline Bovard was stationed, or to Madigan U.S. Army Medical Center. The request for transfer to Madigan Medical Center was approved by the Surgeon General.

Jun 1995 Brig. Gen. Nancy R. Adams participated in the groundbreaking for the "Women in the Military Service for America" memorial with President Bill Clinton. This is the first national memorial commemorating the contributions and achievements of all military women, in all wars, all grades, and all periods of time.

27 Jul 1995 The Korean War Veterans Monument was dedicated in Washington, D.C. The monument is a tribute to veterans of the Korean War and their deceased and MIA comrades.

Printed in the United States
208430BV00001B/93/A

9 780898 754933